4th Edition

ATI TEAS® 7
CRASH COURSE®

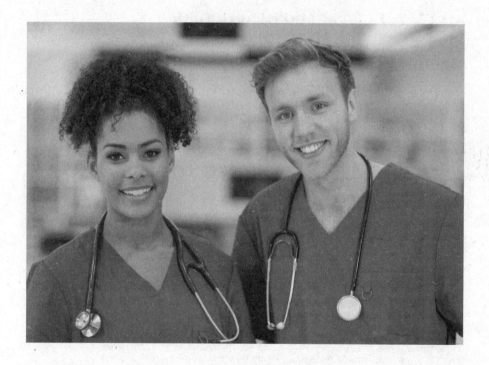

John Allen

T0002830

Research & Education Association
www.rea.com

Research & Education Association
1325 Franklin Ave., Suite 250
Garden City, NY 11530
Email: info@rea.com

ATI TEAS® 7 CRASH COURSE,® 4th Edition

Printed in the United States of America

Library of Congress Control Number 2023948260

ISBN-13: 978-0-7386-1284-3
ISBN-10: 0-7386-1284-7

HB 10 19 2023 1233

TABLE of CONTENTS

ABOUT THIS BOOK

REA's *ATI TEAS 7 Crash Course* is an essential guide for the time-crunched nursing school or allied health program applicant who wants a quick refresher before taking Version 7 of the Test of Essential Academic Skills, or TEAS. It offers a preview of the content found on the most recent version of the exam.

This *Crash Course* includes review chapters specifically targeted to what you need to know to ace the exam. Each skill objective is concisely covered, with one or more practice questions included to test your comprehension. The format of the *ATI TEAS 7 Crash Course* makes it easy to focus on the specific skills where you need the most review.

Chapter 1 describes the format and content of the TEAS, including important changes reflected in the current exam. It also includes proven test-taking strategies and a discussion of the personal qualities needed to succeed in the nursing profession.

Chapters 2 through 5 provide tightly focused skill reviews on Reading, Mathematics, Science, and English and Language Usage. Each skill objective is covered separately, with bulleted items that describe what you need to know about the skill. The sample questions at the end of each section offer practice in the multiple-choice format you will see on the TEAS.

REA's *ATI TEAS 7 Crash Course* will help you build your confidence as you review the various topics and skills. This book will show you how to study efficiently and strategically, so you can earn a high score on this important exam.

Good luck on the TEAS 7!

To check your test readiness for the TEAS 7, either before or after studying this *Crash Course*, take REA's **online practice exam**. To access your practice exam, visit the online REA Study Center at *www.rea.com/studycenter* and follow the on-screen instructions. This true-to-format test features automatic scoring, detailed answer explanations, and diagnostic score reporting that will help you identify your strengths and weaknesses so you'll be ready for test day.

A NOTE FROM OUR AUTHOR

The basic approach of this *ATI TEAS 7 Crash Course* is simple: the targeted content review covers exactly what you need to know for Version 7 of the TEAS exam. You can proceed to the topics you most need to study without slogging through long paragraphs and complicated explanations. The sample problems in the book demonstrate the strategies you should use in answering the types of questions you will see on the TEAS.

Before you begin studying, ask yourself how prepared you are to take the TEAS. Some students are ready to take the test as soon as they pick up this book, while others may be completely unprepared. Most test-takers will fall somewhere in between. Most likely, you're more confident—and competent—in some areas than in others. So what should you do? Here are four ways to study using this *Crash Course*. Pick the one that suits your situation the best.

- **The Systematic Approach:** Start at the beginning and go through the entire book, chapter by chapter, section by section, and make sure you cover every topic thoroughly.

- **The Strength Approach:** Review the sections that you feel are your strong points, then go on to areas that give you trouble. Starting with your strengths will give you confidence and make you familiar with the book's format. Then you can tackle your problem areas with a positive attitude and, ultimately, do well on the test.

- **The Weakness Approach:** Concentrate on the sections you feel are your weakest and move on from there. For example, are your math skills rusty? Then start with Chapter 3 and study it carefully. Once you have shored up your weak areas, you can move on to your stronger areas, building your knowledge and confidence section by section.

- **The Blank Slate Approach:** Are you unsure of your strengths and weaknesses in basic academic skills? Then start anywhere in the book and branch out from there. As you review each section, you'll soon get an idea of how much you know (or don't know) about a given topic. This will tell you what you need to go over a second or a third time. You'll end by gaining knowledge and a strong belief in yourself.

Whichever approach you use, you will eventually reach the point where you are ready to take a practice test. Go to the online REA Study Center at *www.rea.com/studycenter,* take the full-length TEAS 7 practice test, and see how well you score. (You can also take the online practice test *before* you begin studying this guide to gauge your overall understanding of the topics tested on the TEAS.) Topic-level score reports will pinpoint your strengths and weaknesses and show you where you need further review.

If after taking REA's online practice exam, you want even more TEAS prep, you can also obtain additional practice using the ATI (Assessment Technologies Institute) online test banks. You can also purchase the official ATI TEAS Study Manual at *https://atitesting.com.*

Study hard, and good luck on your test!

—*John Allen*

ABOUT OUR AUTHOR

John Allen is a veteran test prep author. Mr. Allen received his B.A. from the University of Oklahoma. He has written many textbooks in the subject areas of English language arts, reading, mathematics, science, and history.

ACKNOWLEDGMENTS

We would like to thank Pam Weston, Publisher, for setting the quality standards for production integrity and managing the publication to completion; Larry B. Kling, Editorial Director, for supervision of revisions and overall direction; Fiona Hallowell for proofreading; Heidi Gagnon for digital file prep; Jennifer Calhoun for page design, revision, and file prep; and Kathy Caratozzolo of Caragraphics for typesetting.

ABOUT REA

Founded in 1959, Research & Education Association (REA) is dedicated to publishing the finest and most effective educational materials—including study guides and test preps—for students of all ages.

Today, REA's wide-ranging catalog is a leading resource for students, teachers, and other professionals. Visit *www.rea.com* to see our complete catalog.

GETTING STARTED

TEAS 7 OVERVIEW

The ATI Test of Essential Academic Skills (TEAS) is designed to assess a student's academic readiness for nursing school and allied health programs in the United States. The TEAS helps predict the performance of incoming candidates and also lets educators learn more about the strengths of admitted students.

In June 2022, the test creator, Assessment Technologies Institute (ATI), replaced the TEAS 6 with the new TEAS Version 7. The revision ensures that the exam meets current standards for nursing and allied health education. There is no content difference between the TEAS for Nursing and the TEAS for Allied Health; just the score reports and official transcripts are different.

While there is no universal passing score for the TEAS, a competitive composite score is viewed as being in the range of 70% to 75%, according to ATI. Nonetheless, you should consult your program about its score requirements.

The TEAS 7 is given in two formats: paper-and-pencil and computer-based. The paper-and-pencil version features only multiple-choice questions. The computerized format features multiple-choice, multiple-correct, supply-answer (fill-in-the-blank), hot-spot, and ordered-response questions.

The TEAS 7 is divided into four separately timed main content areas: Reading, Mathematics, Science, and English and Language Usage. The exam has 170 test items, 20 of which are not scored, making a total of 150 scored items. You will have 209 minutes to take the test. The exam lets you review your work within any of the four active sections (Reading, Math, Science, and English and Language Usage). Once you close a section, however, you cannot go back.

TEAS 7 EXAM AT A GLANCE

Content Area	Number of Questions	Time Limit	Estimated Time Per Question
Reading	45	55 minutes	1.2 minutes
Mathematics	38	57 minutes	1.5 minutes
Science	50	60 minutes	1.2 minutes
English and Language Usage	37	37 minutes	1 minute
Total	**170**	**209 minutes**	

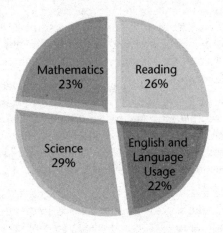

Every content area is divided into sub-content areas, each of which has a specific number of scored items on the test. (The unscored items are being researched for possible inclusion in future editions of the TEAS.) Some of the sub-content areas for TEAS 7 are new. In the Science section, biology and chemistry receive more emphasis. For English and Language Usage, the test places added focus on how language and vocabulary are used to put ideas in writing. Here's a breakdown at the subcategory level of the exam, including the approximate percentage of the main content areas and subcategories:

TEAS EXAM SUBCATEGORIES

Content and Subcategories	Approx. Percent of Exam/Section
Reading	26%
Key Ideas and Details	10%
Craft and Structure	6%
Integration of Knowledge and Ideas	10%
Mathematics	23%
Numbers and Algebra	12%
Measurement and Data	11%
Science	29%
Human Anatomy and Physiology	12%
Biology	6%
Chemistry	5%
Scientific Reasoning	6%
English and Language Usage	22%
Conventions of Standard English	8%
Knowledge of Language	7%
Using Language and Vocabulary to Express Ideas in Writing	7%

REGISTERING FOR THE EXAM

Before you can register for the TEAS, you must create an account at the ATI testing website, *www.atitesting.com*. Once your account is set up, you can view more information about the registration process, fees, payment options, and score reports. You may choose between in-person and remote-proctoring options that allow you to take the test from home. Learn more at *https://www.atitesting.com/teas/exam-details*.

It costs about $120 to take the TEAS. Other cost variables apart from the exam fee include proctoring fees, scheduling fees, security monitoring fees for remote exams, etc.

Once you've registered, you will receive a receipt/confirmation email from ATI containing the ID number required to complete scheduling of the test.

Keep in mind that there is a no-refund policy on TEAS registration. When you register at *www.atitesting.com*, all registrations are final. If you're unable to attend the scheduled test date, you must re-register and pay for a new exam date.

Accommodations for individuals with documented disabilities may be available under the Americans with Disabilities Act.

Check with your nursing or allied health program for specific scoring and entrance requirements regarding the TEAS. You should also consult your program's policy on retaking the TEAS. Should you need to retake the exam, you may not retake any one section. Candidates must complete all four sections of the TEAS at any sitting.

CAN I USE A CALCULATOR ON THE TEAS?

Yes. The TEAS allows for the use of a four-function calculator. Do not bring your own calculator to the testing center, as an on-screen calculator is embedded within the online version of the exam. For the paper-and-pencil version of the TEAS, the testing center will provide you with a four-function calculator.

WHAT TO BRING TO THE TEST (AND WHAT NOT TO BRING)

Be sure to bring:

Valid photo identification of yourself, such as a driver's license, passport, or Green Card (formally known as a Permanent Resident Card). To be admitted to the test, your ID must be government-issued and have a current photograph, your permanent address, and your signature. A photo credit card or student ID are not sufficient to meet the criteria for admission to the test center.

If you're taking the paper-and-pencil version of the exam, be sure to bring two sharpened No. 2 pencils with erasers. No other writing utensils are allowed. Calculators will be provided for certain sections of the TEAS.

If you're taking the online version of the test, you must bring your login information with you. Your student account must be created beforehand at *www.atitesting.com* prior to the day of the test.

Do not bring:

Additional clothing, including jackets, coats, and hats. All clothing is subject to inspection by the test proctor. (Allowances may be made for religious apparel.)

Personal items of any kind, such as purses, backpacks, duffel bags, and computer cases.

Electronic devices of any kind, including cellphones, smartphones, beepers/pagers, and digital watches.

Food or drink, unless you have a documented medical need for such an item.

PREPARING FOR NEW QUESTION TYPES

Computer-based versions of the TEAS 7 exam feature four so-called alternate question types in addition to the standard multiple-choice questions you're likely familiar with. They include the following:

Multiple-select questions give you four or more answer choices, of which more than one answer choice may be correct. For these questions a prompt will appear telling you to "select all that apply." To answer a multiple-select question correctly, you must choose all the answers that are correct. No partial credit is given.

- There's a bit of a twist to watch for: Even though they're named multiple-select questions, there may be cases where there is only one correct answer, while, on the other hand, in certain cases, all answer choices could be correct. Evaluate each answer choice individually.

Supply-answer questions ask you to fill in the blank or supply the correct answer yourself. No answer choices are provided.

- To check your answer to a supply-answer question, re-read the entire sentence with your fill-in-the-blank response to see if it makes sense.

Hot-spot questions require you to click on the area of an image that correctly answers the question. Each image will contain from two to five clickable areas for your response.

- Before making your choice, look carefully at each clickable area on the image. Remember that only one clickable area is correct.

Ordered-response questions require you to put a set of given elements in the correct order. You do this by dragging each item from a box on the left to its correct place in a box on the right. If any item is out of order, the entire question is incorrect.

- After you have placed the items in order, check the sequence carefully from beginning to end.

GENERAL TEST-TAKING STRATEGIES FOR THE TEAS

Answer every question. You won't be penalized for wrong answers, so make sure you answer every question, even if you guess.

Make an educated guess. An educated guess—when you have some idea about the correct answer—is a much better choice than an uneducated "wild" guess, in which you randomly choose an answer. When dealing with standard four-choice multiple-choice items, informed guesses can help you tilt the odds in your favor:

- With an "uneducated" guess, in which your answer choice is random, your answer has a 25% chance of being correct.

- If you can eliminate one wrong answer, your guess has a 33% chance of being correct.

- If you can eliminate two wrong answers, your guess has a 50% chance of being correct.

Answer the easy questions first. Don't worry about answering questions in order. Look for questions you know first. This allows you to move ahead on the test and then come back to the more difficult questions and give them more thought.

Mark the tough questions. If a question strikes you as troublesome, ambiguous, or for some reason too hard to answer, mark it and come back to it later. Likewise, if you have an answer that you're unsure of, mark it for review as well.

Be aware of the clock. Keep in mind how much time you have for each test section. For example, you will have 55 minutes to complete the Reading section of the test. After 15 minutes, you should have answered about 11 to 13 of the 45 Reading questions. After a half hour, you should have answered about 22 to 26 of the Reading questions, and so forth.

Aim to have spare time after you have gone through the entire test. Your goal should be to complete the test with at least 10 minutes to spare. This will give you time to go over the most difficult questions that you had trouble answering. However, if you don't reach your goal of leaving spare time at the end of the test, don't worry. The most important time management element is to stay calm, work steadily, and answer all the questions.

Be intuitive. In general, your first guess at a question you don't know is often your best guess. If an answer *seems* better, it often is.

Identify what is being asked. Your first order of business for a question is to make sure you are answering what is actually being asked. For example, look at the units of the answer for gas mileage. If your answer is not in miles per gallon, it can't be correct.

Watch out for decoy answers. Most questions have one or two wrong answers that are way off the mark and at least one answer that is plausible in some way.

- Eliminate the clearly wrong answers right away.

- Then consider the two or three plausible answers remaining. Try plugging these answers back into the question to see if they make sense.

- If you still can't identify the best answer, use your intuition to make an educated guess.

Review your answer. Work as quickly as possible but always take time to review the answer that you choose. Ask yourself:

- Does this answer make sense?

- Am I falling for a decoy (aka a distractor)?

- Did I find the answer that the problem was actually asking for?

Stay calm. Stressing out over the test makes your results worse, not better. So focus on serenity. Think of your stress as an energy source that can be harnessed and used in a positive rather than a negative way.

Avoid these mistakes in preparing for the test:

- **Failing to eat a good breakfast.** Your brain needs to be in top working order during the test. You can't afford to run out of energy or lose focus. Try to eat well and sleep well as you prepare for the test.

- **Overconfidence.** If you are a qualified applicant, the TEAS should not seem overly difficult. However, you shouldn't take the test lightly either. Be serious. Give the test the respect it deserves. Your nursing career may depend on it.

- **A bad attitude.** You may consider yourself a poor test-taker, but apprehension, fear, and pessimism can only make your performance worse. Try to approach the test with an air of quiet confidence.

- **Cramming.** You may be able to cram for a narrowly focused junior high spelling test, but the TEAS is too broad, too varied, and too general for last-minute cramming. Cramming can only result in making you tired and anxious on exam day.

Follow these smart tips that lead to success on the test:

- **Get regular exercise.** Exercise does more than build physical stamina; it also builds mental endurance. You will need plenty of both kinds of stamina when taking the test. Get into an exercise routine weeks before you take the test. You will eat better, sleep better, and study more effectively as a result.

- **Get help.** Don't know much about chemistry? Rather than try to learn it all on your own, seek out someone who can help—a friend, sibling, teacher, tutor, or parent.

- **Set goals.** The key to getting things done is to map out your study goals ahead of time. Chart your progress on a table or graph.

- **Be honest with yourself.** If you're not good with fractions, it won't help to skip over them and hope they don't show up on the test. Realistically assess your strengths and weaknesses. Work extra hard on the skills that give you trouble.

SETTING UP A STUDY PLAN

First, determine how much time you have before the test and how much time you can realistically devote to preparation each day. Do you have months? Weeks? Only a few days? The amount of study time you have will determine how your study plan proceeds.

Find your strengths and weaknesses. (This is precisely where taking REA's online practice test will come in handy.) Then find those topics in this book and work on them. Look at the following chart as an example.

SELF-EVALUATION CHART

	I'm confident	I need to review	When I studied
Reading			
Summarizing			
Make inferences and draw conclusions			
Identify topic, main idea, and supporting details			
Follow written directions			
Find specific information in a text			
Analyze and interpret information from graphics			
Recognize sequence			
Distinguish between fact and opinion			
Text structure			
Context clues			
Author's purpose			
Author's point of view			
Text features			
Make predictions and draw conclusions			
Compare themes			
Evaluate an argument			
Integrate data from multiple sources			
Mathematics			
Fractions, decimals, and percentages			
Perform operations with rational numbers			
Compare and order rational numbers			
Solve equations in one variable			
Solve real-world problems with rational numbers			
Solve real-world problems with percentages			

(continued)

	I'm confident	I need to review	When I studied
Estimation and rounding			
Proportions			
Ratios and rates of change			
Solve real-world problems with expressions, equations, and inequalities			
Tables, charts, and graphs			
Evaluate information in data sets			
Relationship between two variables			
Calculate geometric quantities			
Standard and metric systems			
Science			
General human anatomy			
Body systems			
Macromolecules			
Cell structure and function			
Mitosis and meiosis			
Microorganisms and infectious disease			
Chromosomes, genes, and DNA			
Mendel's laws of heredity			
Atomic structure			
Properties of substances			
Changes in states of matter			
Chemical reactions			
Properties of solutions			
Acids and bases			
Scientific measurements and tools			
Apply logic and evidence to a scientific explanation			
Predict relationships			
Design of a scientific investigation			

(continued)

	I'm confident	I need to review	When I studied
English and Language Usage			
Spelling			
Punctuation			
Sentence structures			
Use grammar for clarity			
Formal and informal language			
Develop a well-organized paragraph			
Apply knowledge of the writing process			
Word-part analysis to determine meaning			

Set up a calendar on which you schedule various study areas and mark off how much time you spend on them in the chart above.

An alternative strategy, especially if you have a lot of time, involves working systematically through this entire book from start to finish. You should find the review to be extremely helpful, and you will be surprised at how many new things you learn even in areas in which you previously thought you were strong.

Use triage at all times. If you have only a few weeks to prepare, you need to focus only on weaknesses and general areas. You don't have time to be systematic. On the other hand, if your time is not limited and you find that spending extra time on a topic such as macromolecules is valuable, go ahead and do it.

Establish a regular study time and try not to let anything interfere with it. Remember, the work you put in now for this test has the promise of paying off over a lifetime.

TEST STRATEGIES FOR SPECIFIC QUESTION TYPES

READING COMPREHENSION PASSAGES

One of the common question types on the TEAS is the long reading passage from which you'll need to draw conclusions and make judgments about things like author's purpose.

Read the title and scan the paragraphs. Get a feel for what the topic is and what to expect from your reading. Note whether multiple questions are associated with the passage. In many cases, they will be.

After previewing the title and general text structure, many fluent test-takers like to go over the questions before they read the passage. Note: This technique may or may not be for you! However, if you are a person who benefits from a question preview, go ahead and do it.

Read quickly but carefully. After each section, briefly review what you just read before you continue. After finishing, consider the piece as a whole. How did the paragraphs fit together? What was the main point of the piece? How was it supported?

Feel free to underline, circle, and write notes as you read. For example, if you view a sentence as providing critical support for a key idea within the passage, mark it clearly.

Finish the passage and go on to the questions. If the first question or two seem daunting, keep moving until you come to a question you are sure of. Then go back to the more difficult questions.

MATH WORD PROBLEMS AND PROBLEM SOLVING

The TEAS Mathematics section has many different types of word problems. Some are simple and require only a quick calculation. Others are complex and may require a detailed analysis. For any word problem, whether it involves whole numbers, fractions, algebra, or any of the topics in Chapter 3, follow these basic steps.

Problem Solving: Basic Steps

1. **Read the problem carefully.** Many problems are misunderstood simply because the problem solver fails to understand the situation fully.

2. **If possible, solve immediately.** If you see the key relationship right away, there is no need to go through a complex analysis. Solve. Then go on to step 7 below.

3. **Underline, circle, write, list.** If you don't see the key relationship right away, mark up the problem by circling, underlining, or making lists and writing equations as befits the version of the test you're taking: online or paper-based. You

may wish to list information in two sections that roughly set out "What I know" versus "What I don't know."

4. **Identify what you need to find.** This is usually the most important step in the process. Find out what you need to know. Focus on the units of your unknown such as inches, grams, milliliters, or miles per hour.

5. **Make a plan.** For simple problems, this might entail nothing more than identifying an operation—addition, subtraction, multiplication, or division—to carry out. For more complex problems, your plan may involve more than one step and more than one operation. In your plan, look for **key words**.

Add +	Subtract −	Multiply ×	Divide ÷
▪ in all	▪ less than	▪ product of	▪ quotient
▪ sum	▪ fewer than	▪ times	▪ per
▪ total	▪ more than	▪ multiplied by	▪ each
▪ together	▪ minus	▪ increased by	▪ equal parts
▪ sum total	▪ difference	▪ a factor of	▪ split
▪ combined	▪ take away		▪ divided by
▪ plus	▪ left over		▪ ratio of
	▪ decreased by		
	▪ increased by		

6. **Set up the problem and solve.** Carry out your plan and calculate the answer.

7. **Go over your answer.** First ask, "Did I find what I was looking for?" If you were looking for miles per gallon and you found gallons per mile, your answer is almost certainly wrong. Check your units. Check your calculations. Make sure that your answer solves the problem.

PROBLEM-SOLVING DO'S AND DON'TS

 DO

- **Write.** Writing things out helps you visualize the problem. Also draw, diagram, model—do anything that helps you see relationships.

- **Estimate.** Use estimation both before and after you solve the problem. Preview to estimate what your answer should be; then check to see whether your answer was correct.

- **Ask yourself, "Does this make sense?"** This is probably the most important step after you've solved the problem. Does your final answer fit the situation and seem reasonable for the context? If not, it's probably best to rethink the problem.

- **Think simple.** The test is not out to force you to make complicated and "messy" calculations. If you get an answer that seems overly jumbled or complicated, it's probably wrong.

 DON'T

- **Try to do it in your head.** Mental math and estimation work only with simple relationships and simple numbers. If you have any doubt, write out the problem. Being able to see your thought process on paper is always a good check.

- **Jump to conclusions.** Make sure you understand what the problem is asking for before you answer it.

- **Rush.** The worst thing about rushing is that it makes you sloppy and careless. Press ahead but always focus on staying calm and steady.

- **Be stubborn.** Being sure you're right is good. Being *too* sure is not good. If your problem-solving procedure or your answer seems suspect, don't hesitate to rethink the problem and start all over.

GRAMMAR-QUESTION TYPE: WHICH SENTENCE IS WRITTEN CORRECTLY?

One of the most common—and most important—question types in the English and Language Usage section of the TEAS essentially asks, "Which sentence is written correctly?"

1. **Look for obvious mistakes.** Questions might include such errors as failing to capitalize the first word in the sentence, misplaced apostrophes, or failing to put punctuation at the end of the sentence.

2. **Is the sentence complete?** Answer choices may feature dependent clauses or other nonsentences trying to pass as sentences. Make sure that the sentence has a complete subject and complete predicate and is not a dependent clause. For example:

   After the rain stopped in the meadow. (Not a complete sentence)

   After the rain stopped in the meadow, we ate lunch. (Complete sentence)

3. **Do the subject and verb agree?** Examples:

   Is Mary and John interested in lunch? (Incorrect)

   Are Mary and John interested in lunch? (Correct)

4. **Are there pronoun or possessive errors?** Objective and subjective cases should not be confused.

   Bob gave advice to Mary and I. (Incorrect)

   Bob gave advice to Mary and me. (Correct)

   Everyone should keep their room clean. (Incorrect)

   Everyone should keep his or her room clean. (Correct)

5. **Should the sentence be broken up?** Test questions often feature run-on sentences that should be broken into two sentences:

   Bob is hungry Mary is not hungry. (Incorrect)

   Bob is hungry. Mary is not hungry. (Correct)

6. **Are there comma errors?** Comma errors include commas in a series; comma splices, which incorrectly join two independent clauses; and failure to insert commas with coordinating conjunctions and dependent clauses.

   Bob is hungry, Mary is nervous. (Incorrect; comma splice)

   Bob is hungry. Mary is nervous. (Correct)

   John ate rice beans and salsa. (Incorrect)

   John ate rice, beans, and salsa. (Correct)

   Bob was hungry so Mary gave him a bagel. (Incorrect)

Bob was hungry, so Mary gave him a bagel. (Correct)

After dinner we went for a walk. (Incorrect)

After dinner, we went for a walk. (Correct)

7. **Are there spelling errors?** Look for commonly confused words, such as *effect* versus *affect* or *accept* versus *except*.

8. **Is the sentence unclear or ambiguous?** Focus on making sure that the sentence conveys its intended message.

Evita wore her yellow dress on the beach that was breathtakingly beautiful. (Unclear: What was "breathtakingly beautiful," the dress or the beach?)

On a breathtakingly beautiful beach, Evita wore her yellow dress. (Clear)

SCIENCE GRAPHICS: INTERPRETING GRAPHS, CHARTS, AND OTHER GRAPHICS

The Science section of the TEAS presents graphs, charts, and other types of visual images. Make sure you understand what each question wants you to do with the information in the accompanying graphic.

Identification. TEAS science questions may not ask for analysis; you may only have to identify a familiar graphic. For example, you might need to identify a diagram of a particular body system.

Types of graphics. Be aware of how different types of graphics present information in different ways. For example, line graphs and bar graphs show relationships. Make sure you identify each axis of the graph and understand what the graph is showing.

Trends. A graph-based question may ask you to identify trends shown in the graph. For example, you may be asked to compare the solubility of two different substances in water as the temperature rises. Your task is to identify the trend—increasing? decreasing?—for each substance.

Drawing conclusions vs. extracting data. Make sure you understand what the question is asking for. Many graphic-based questions ask you to draw a conclusion: Which is greater? What change do you see? Other questions require you to extract information: Which chamber of the heart pumps the blood to the lungs?

IS NURSING (OR ALLIED HEALTH) FOR YOU?

Before settling on nursing or allied health as a career, ask yourself the following questions:

- Are you a compassionate, empathetic, caring person?

- How well do you deal with stress?

- How good are you at following directions?

- How comfortable are you with a job that presents new challenges every day rather than the security of knowing what you are going to do every day?

- How comfortable are you working with and serving people of all kinds of ethnicities and backgrounds?

- How comfortable are you in dealing with sickness, pain, and the end of life?

- How squeamish are you with regard to the most basic and "messy" human functions, both physical and psychological?

- Are you a good team player?

- How comfortable are you in dealing with difficult and even abusive people?

- How good are you at admitting mistakes, learning from mistakes, and forgiving mistakes in others?

- How good are you at critical thinking? Are you comfortable in expressing your point of view even in the face of strong resistance?

- How responsible, reliable, and punctual are you?

- How comfortable are you in following orders and directions even when they may be flawed?

What kind of nurse do you want to be? There are four types of nursing degrees:

- An Associate's Degree in Nursing (ADN) is issued by 2-year schools.

- A Bachelor's Degree in Nursing (BSN) is issued by a 4-year college or university.

- A Master's Degree in Nursing (MSN) is obtained after completing a BSN and requires completing a graduate master's program.

- A doctorate in nursing is the highest degree obtainable and focuses on the most advanced and analytical aspects of the nursing profession.

Nursing levels include the following:

- A Licensed Practical Nurse (LPN) or a Licensed Vocational Nurse (LVN) has completed only 1 year of post-high school nursing education.

- A Registered Nurse (RN) must have at least an ADN and typically requires a BSN. RNs must also pass a licensing test to practice.

- Advanced categories for nursing include such things as Nurse Practitioner (NP) or Clinical Nurse Specialist (CNS).

In becoming a nurse, you will need to choose:

- Medical specialty: e.g., surgery, OB/GYN, gastroenterology, emergency

- Where you work: e.g., hospital, clinic, doctor's office, school, military base, private practice, hospice, government agency

- Nursing specialties include nurse anesthetist, nurse midwife, nurse administrator, home health nurse, general duty nurse

READING

The first section of the TEAS covers Reading. It features 39 scored items. There are three categories of Reading objectives for the TEAS. The test items are divided among the Reading objectives as follows.

R.1 KEY IDEAS AND DETAILS—15 SCORED QUESTIONS

R.1.1   Summarize a complex text.

R.1.2   Infer the logical conclusion from a reading selection.

R.1.3   Identify the topic, main idea, and supporting details.

R.1.4   Follow a given set of directions.

R.1.5   Identify specific information from a printed communication.

R.1.6   Analyze and interpret information from a graphic.

R.1.7   Recognize events in a sequence.

R.2 CRAFT AND STRUCTURE—9 SCORED QUESTIONS

R.2.1   Distinguish between fact and opinion, biases, and stereotypes.

R.2.2   Recognize the structure of texts in various formats.

R.2.3   Interpret the meaning of words and phrases using context.

R.2.4   Evaluate the author's purpose in a given text.

R.2.5   Evaluate the author's point of view in a given text.

R.2.6   Use text features.

R.3 INTEGRATION OF KNOWLEDGE AND IDEAS—15 SCORED QUESTIONS

R.3.1   Identify primary sources in various media.

R.3.2   Use evidence from text to make predictions and inferences, and draw conclusions about a piece of writing.

R.3.3   Compare and contrast themes from print and other sources.

R.3.4   Evaluate an argument and its specific claims.

R.3.5   Evaluate and integrate data from multiple sources.

The TEAS Reading section also features six unscored items (aka "pretest" items). These items can address objectives from any of the above categories. You will have 55 minutes to complete the entire Reading section.

The TEAS Reading section includes reading passages from different genres, both fiction and nonfiction. A single reading passage may be followed by several questions that refer to the passage and cover different skills. You should read each passage carefully and refer to it as you answer the questions.

R. 1. KEY IDEAS AND DETAILS

R.1.1 SUMMARIZE A COMPLEX TEXT

A good way to demonstrate text comprehension is to summarize the passage you're given. You must be able to identify the topic of the text, what the text tells about the topic, and why this information is important. Here's how:

First, look for the topic, which is the overall subject of the text. It can be expressed as a word or phrase. Some examples of topics are placebos, jogging, tropical fish, alternative energy, and meteorites. To find the topic of a text, ask yourself, "What is this passage about?"

Next, you should identify what information the text provides about the topic. This is the focus of the passage. For example, the text might explain how placebos are tested or where meteorites come from. You should identify important points that the writer supplies about the topic.

Finally, you should look for the main idea or key point the writer is making about the topic. The writer might be making a case for more frequent use of placebos. She might be explaining what meteorites can tell us about the chemical makeup of other planets.

Sometimes the summary of a text can be found in the first sentence or two. An opening sentence might say:

> The development of alternative sources of energy benefits society in many ways.

The topic is alternative sources of energy. The key point is that developing these sources benefits society in many ways.

When you summarize a complex text, you rephrase it in shorter form, focusing on the topic and main ideas.

On the Reading portion of the TEAS exam you will not actually summarize a complex text in your own words. Instead you will answer multiple-choice questions in which you choose the best summary of the text or the best statement of the main idea. For this skill, the TEAS includes questions like these:

- Which of the following best expresses the key point of this passage?

- In this passage, the writer's main concern is to discuss which of the following?

- Which best describes the overall topic of this passage?

R.1.1 PROBLEM

Read the following passage. Then answer the question.

Science fiction explores a number of themes repeatedly. One popular theme that presents many fascinating possibilities is time travel. Charles Dickens had his miserly character Ebenezer Scrooge reexamine his life by traveling back to the past and forward to a chilling future. Mark Twain sent his Connecticut Yankee back in time to have adventures at King Arthur's court. These time travels were accomplished through dreams and fantasy. In his 1895 novel *The Time Machine,* H.G. Wells depicted time travel by mechanical means. Later authors imagined how time travelers might alter the present by changing the past. John Buchan's novel *The Gap in the Curtain* presents a group of people whose lives are disrupted when they read a newspaper item from the future. Today's science fiction writers also employ time travel as a plot device, often with an emphasis on details from modern physics.

Which of the following best expresses the key point of this passage?

(A) Charles Dickens, Mark Twain, and H.G. Wells employed many of the same themes in their writing.

(B) Time travel is a popular theme of science fiction that many writers, both past and present, have used in fascinating ways.

(C) Science fiction writers tend to explore a number of themes over and over.

(D) Time travel is the most fascinating theme available to science fiction writers who understand modern physics.

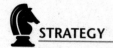

STRATEGY

Summarizing requires a reader to distill and condense a text into its most basic form, stripping away all inessential items and leaving just the most critical information. Look for the answer that best summarizes the main idea of the passage.

THINK

- The first sentence of this text does not provide a summary of the passage. The main point of the passage begins with the second sentence, about time travel as a popular theme for science fiction.

- (A) is incorrect because the passage is not about the various themes used by these writers.

- (C) is incorrect because it doesn't mention time travel as a science fiction theme.

- (D) is incorrect because it focuses only on the last sentence. The correct answer is (B).

R.1.2 INFER THE LOGICAL CONCLUSION FROM A READING SELECTION

To show comprehension of a text—which could be a story, news article, information piece, or blog post—the reader must make inferences about what the text means. An inference is a conclusion based on critical thinking skills. To infer something from a text is to read between the lines and decide what the text means. A good reader approaches a reading selection like a detective looking for evidence.

- Look for clues about meaning, such as key terms, descriptive details, emotional words, value judgments, and overall tone.

- Try to distinguish facts from opinions and decide what is valid.

- Draw upon your own experience in evaluating a reading selection. Perhaps it describes a situation that's familiar to you. This prior knowledge can help you make a correct inference or draw a logical conclusion about what is happening or what the passage means.

Instead of stating things outright, writers often provide clues and details that allow the reader to infer what is going on in the text. For example, you might read an article about events that took place in a hospital. The article describes a snowstorm occurring that afternoon. You can make the assumption that the events took place during the winter months. Of course, your inference may be incorrect. As you read, look for additional clues to confirm or disprove your reasoned hunch.

The reader should also look for words that show a sequence of events or chronology, as well as words that describe emotions or make value judgments. Look at this example:

> The next time the owner of the pastry shop saw Stanley at the door, she quickly slipped a plate of sample cupcakes under the counter. The smile she gave Stanley was wonderfully fake.

The reader can infer that the owner recognizes Stanley from a previous visit and moves the sample cupcakes so that he will not eat them. The owner's fake smile indicates she does not like Stanley.

When you infer the logical conclusion from a text, you use details from the passage along with your own prior knowledge and experience to decide what the passage means or what the author is trying to say.

The Reading section of the TEAS exam will also require you to draw a conclusion about a passage. Drawing a conclusion is slightly different from making an inference. When you draw a conclusion, you make an overall judgment based on details, personal knowledge, and inferences. Look at this example:

> Joseph held strong opinions about the Vietnam War, which lasted from 1954 to 1975. He came from a military family, whose members had seen combat in several wars. He himself enlisted in the Marines in 1978 at the age of nineteen. Joseph's impressions of how Vietnam affected military culture in the United States make for powerful reading.

From details in the passage, you can draw the conclusion that Joseph did not see combat in Vietnam. The war was over by the time he joined the military.

R.1.2 PROBLEM

Read the following passage. Then answer the question.

It has become fashionable in certain circles to deny that William Shakespeare wrote Shakespeare's plays. Some insist, with a shaky grasp of the historical record, that the Bard never attended school and could barely even write his own name. They believe his only connection to the plays was to serve as a front for the real genius, a shy type who apparently preferred to stay in the shadows. So who was the genuine writer? Some say it was Sir Francis Bacon, others put the finger on the Earl of Oxford. A few of the unhinged go with Queen Elizabeth herself. For, as everyone knows, you can't write great literature if you don't come from the court or the upper classes. Or so say the anti-Shakespearean snobs.

Which of the following can you infer from the passage?

(A) The writer believes that Shakespeare was a shy person who preferred to stay in the shadows and let others receive credit for his plays.

(B) The writer agrees that only someone from the upper classes could have written Shakespeare's plays.

(C) The writer is uncertain about who is the true author of Shakespeare's plays.

(D) The writer has a low opinion of those who do not believe that William Shakespeare wrote Shakespeare's plays.

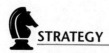

STRATEGY

Look for details about the author's point of view to make inferences about the passage.

THINK

- The writer notes that it is "fashionable" to question Shakespeare's authorship, indicating it is a shallow idea with little substance.

- The writer uses sarcasm and also suggests that the Shakespeare doubters have a "shaky grasp of the historical record," that some are "unhinged," and that they are "anti-Shakespearean snobs."

- These details indicate that the writer has a low opinion of the Shakespeare doubters. Choice (D) is the correct answer.

R.1.3 IDENTIFY THE TOPIC, MAIN IDEA, AND SUPPORTING DETAILS

To understand a passage, you must use critical reading skills. These skills allow you to analyze a text, identify its important parts, and see how they fit together to support the author's meaning.

First, identify the topic of the passage. This is the overall subject that the passage discusses or describes. The topic generally is found in a topic sentence, which can be anywhere in the passage. Often the topic sentence is the first sentence of the passage. It may also be the second sentence or the last sentence in the first paragraph.

Second, identify the main idea of the passage. This is the key point that the writer wants to emphasize about the topic. A good topic sentence includes the topic and the main idea.

Third, identify the supporting details in the passage. These are sentences that develop the main idea. They can explain, clarify, compare, or elaborate on the main point.

Although the entire text has a main idea, each paragraph within the text also has its own main idea.

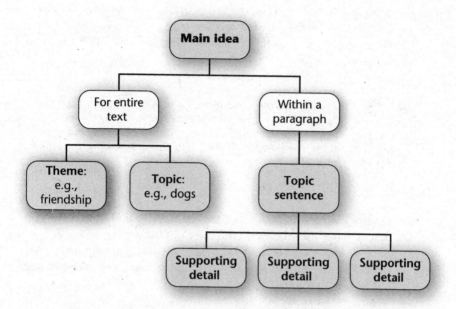

On the TEAS Reading exam, main idea questions are not difficult if you read the passage carefully. Look at the following example:

> When it comes to dieting, Americans tend to make things too difficult. They declare that carbohydrates are the villain and try to avoid them entirely. This is hard to do since carbs are an important source of energy and make up a good portion of a healthy diet. Or they swear off fatty foods and try to live on nuts and berries like an animal in the forest. Some people I know act like the food police when they are around other people. What's needed instead is a back-to-basics approach. A person should eat a well-rounded diet, including vegetables, fruits, meats, and grains. Sweets and oily foods need not be eliminated, only eaten in small amounts. Add a regular exercise regimen and you've got a recipe for a healthy lifestyle.

After reading the passage, ask yourself, "What is the topic?" The answer is "dieting." Then note that the main idea can be found in the first sentence, which is the topic sentence: "Americans tend to make things too difficult." Finally, look for supporting details or sentences that show how Americans make dieting too difficult. One sentence explains how Americans try to avoid carbohydrates entirely. Another says that they swear off fatty foods and try to live on nuts and berries. The last few sentences in the passage present a better approach to dieting that is less difficult and more likely to be successful.

To demonstrate comprehension of a text, you must be able to identify the topic, or what the text is about; the main idea, or the key point the writer makes about the topic; and supporting details, or the points that explain the main idea or add to it.

On the TEAS exam, you might also be asked to find unnecessary details. Note the following sentence from the passage: "Some people I know act like the food police when they are around other people." This sentence does not add to the main idea and thus does not belong in the text.

R.1.3 PROBLEM

Read the following passage. Then answer the question.

Many kinds of sharks are on endangered lists today. This is chiefly due to human activities. Fishing interests hunt sharks for their monetary value and cultural importance. Shark fins are coveted as an ingredient in traditional Chinese medicine. Shark fin soup is valued as a delicacy throughout Asia. Shark finning—the practice of catching sharks, cutting off their fins, and discarding the carcass—is responsible for killing 100 million sharks each year.

Which of the following would be the best addition to this passage?

(A) Fishermen seeking tuna sometimes catch other, non-targeted species in their nets.

(B) Growing demand for shark fins in Hong Kong and elsewhere makes the fin trade extremely lucrative.

(C) Overfishing is an issue that environmental groups are increasingly focused on worldwide.

(D) Mother sharks bear one litter of about eight to twelve babies every other year.

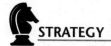

STRATEGY

This question tests whether you can identify relevant supporting details. The correct answer should add to the main idea about why sharks are on endangered lists today.

THINK

- (A) is incorrect because it gives general information about catching non-targeted species.

- (C) is incorrect because it focuses on overfishing in general, not specifically on overfishing for sharks.

- (D) is incorrect because it offers information about how sharks reproduce but does not connect it to the main idea of why sharks are endangered.

- The correct answer is (B).

R.1.4 FOLLOW A GIVEN SET OF DIRECTIONS

Directions or procedural documents are common in daily life. They include instructions for assembly, repair manuals, recipes, workout routines, cellphone procedures, and rules for games.

Nursing and allied health students must follow a set of directions in many areas of study, from lab work to patient care. The TEAS Reading exam requires that you show the ability to follow a set of directions and show how sequential tasks are related.

First, read the entire set of directions carefully. Do not try to carry out the instructions at this point. Look for visual aids such as headings and subheadings, numerical or alphabetical steps, flow charts, diagrams, or photographs.

Next, look for words that indicate sequence or other procedural details.

Follow each step of the directions in sequence.

Finally, when you have finished, go back over the directions to make sure you have followed them correctly and accomplished the overall task.

As you examine a set of directions, look closely for words that signify sequence or order. These include the following:

first	beginning	second	next
now	following	before	after
then	while	finally	last

You should also look for specific terms like left/right, clockwise/counterclockwise, inside/outside, above/below, and top/bottom. Getting one of these wrong can spoil the procedure.

To follow a given set of directions, you should read the directions carefully, note the terms that signify sequence or order, and demonstrate that you understand each step.

R.1.4 PROBLEM

Read the following set of directions. Then answer the question.

1. Start with the words USERS KID.

2. Reverse the order of the words.

3. Insert the letter N after the first vowel in the first word and before the first vowel in the second word.

4. Move the fifth letter in the second word to follow the first vowel in that word.

Which words have you formed?

(A) KIN RUSES (C) INK RUSES

(B) DINK NURSES (D) KIND NURSES

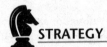

STRATEGY

To find the answer, you must complete the steps in order. Read through the numbered directions completely. Then follow the directions as you go through them a second time.

THINK

- Write the words: USERS KID.

- Reverse the word order: KID USERS.

- Insert N in two places as directed: KI<u>ND</u> <u>N</u>USERS.

- In the second word, move the fifth letter, R, to follow the first vowel, U: KIND NU<u>R</u>SES.

- Write out the words: KIND NURSES. (D) is the correct answer.

R.1.5 IDENTIFY SPECIFIC INFORMATION FROM A PRINTED COMMUNICATION

As a nursing or allied health student, you will encounter many different types of printed communication. Some are technical and formal, such as drug labels and instructions for nursing procedures. Others are more casual, such as staff memos, classified ads, and posted announcements. Printed sources are written to keep you informed and ensure that important information is shared among a group. On the TEAS Reading exam, you must identify and use specific information from these sources.

For memos, posted announcements, and other informal printed communications:

- Identify the intended audience or recipient of the notice. Also identify the source or author of the information.

- Check the date of the notice.

- Identify the subject of the notice.

- Read the information carefully. Look for boldface statements or summary sentences.

For labels, bills, or technical forms:

- Browse the label, bill, or form before you zoom in on the details. Usually it is not necessary to read the whole thing from beginning to end.

- Scan for specific information. For example, on an ingredients list, you might check how many grams of fat a food contains. On a form or bill, you would check to see whether any action or payment is required.

- Check how the label, bill, or form is organized. Specific information may be placed in boxes, rows, or columns. Look for the location of important items or details. The account number of a bill is often in the upper right-hand corner of the first page.

Look for specific information when you examine a printed communication, such as the author or source of the information, its date, its subject, and the way the information is presented or organized.

R.1.5 PROBLEMS

Read the following label of nutrition facts. Then answer the two questions that follow.

Nutrition Facts

Serving Size (343g)
Servings Per Container

Amount Per Serving

Calories 310	Calories from Fat 60

	% Daily Value*
Total Fat 6g	**9%**
Saturated Fat 1g	**5%**
Trans Fat 0g	
Cholesterol 0mg	**0%**
Sodium 70mg	**3%**
Total Carbohydrate 58g	**19%**
Dietary Fiber 7g	**28%**
Sugars 23g	
Protein 5g	

Vitamin A 15%	•	Vitamin C 6%
Calcium 30%	•	Iron 15%

*Percent Daily Values are based on a 2,000 calorie diet. Your daily values may be higher or lower depending on your calorie needs:

	Calories:	2,000	2,500
Total Fat	Less than	65g	80g
Saturated Fat	Less than	20g	25g
Cholesterol	Less than	300mg	300mg
Sodium	Less than	2,400mg	2,400mg
Total Carbohydrate		300g	375g
Dietary Fiber		25g	30g

Calories per gram:
    Fat 9 • Carbohydrate 4 • Protein 4

R.1.5 PROBLEM 1

The doctor has requested that an underweight patient have a high-calorie, low-fat diet. Is this cereal appropriate if it accounts for one-third of his diet?

(A) No, because the cereal is too high in both calories and fat.

(B) No, because the cereal is appropriately low in fat but not high enough in calories.

(C) Yes, because the cereal is appropriately low in fat and appropriately high in calories.

(D) Yes, because the cereal is appropriately high in fat and appropriately low in calories.

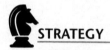 STRATEGY

Read the entire label for clues about the appropriate number of calories and fat that the patient should receive.

THINK

- The label states that the cereal provides 9% of a person's daily recommended fat intake or 6 g of a standard 65 g total for fat. If the cereal represents one-third of the patient's diet, the fat intake from this cereal is low. So with regard to fat, the cereal is appropriate.

- With regard to calories, the cereal provides only 310 calories, far less than the 2,500-calorie diet printed near the bottom of the label. Because the calorie count of the cereal is so low, it is not appropriate.

- Being appropriate for fat but too low for calories matches answer choice (B).

R.1.5 PROBLEM 2

The patient has diabetes, and his doctor recommends that he eat fewer than 200 g of carbohydrate each day. Is this cereal a good choice for the patient who eats three meals a day?

(A) Yes, because the 58 g of carbohydrate represents less than one-third of a 200-g total.

(B) Yes, because the 58 g of carbohydrate represents less than the 200-g total for the day.

(C) No, because the 58 g of carbohydrate represents more than one-third of a 200-g total.

(D) No, because the 58 g of carbohydrate represents far too few carbohydrates per day for a person with diabetes.

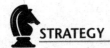 STRATEGY

Because this patient has diabetes, ignore the 300-g recommendation for carbohydrates on the label when evaluating the situation.

THINK

- Assume that the cereal represents one-third of the patient's diet. Multiply the carbohydrate count by 3. If the total exceeds 200 g, then the cereal is not a good choice. If the total is less than 200 g, then the cereal is a good choice.

- 3×58 is equal to 174 g of carbohydrate, well under the limit of 200 g for people with diabetes, so this cereal is a good choice, making answer choice (A) correct. (B) is incorrect because it compares the 58 g with the entire day's 200-g total. (C) is incorrect because the math does not compute, and (D) is incorrect because it makes the irrelevant assertion that the cereal is not appropriate.

R.1.6 ANALYZE AND INTERPRET INFORMATION FROM A GRAPHIC

Graphic representations provide complex information or statistics in the form of a visual summary. They enable the reader to compare numbers, check percentages, follow a sequence, or trace a route. Most graphics feature titles and subheads that explain their purpose. The TEAS Reading exam will test your ability to read a graphic and interpret the information it presents.

Identify what type of graphic it is and think about how to read it. There are many different ways to present information graphically. The most common forms include graphs, charts, tables, maps, and instrument scales.

Visualize the "big picture" that the graphic presents, or assess its overall meaning. If it is a line graph, is it trending up or down? If it is an instrument scale, what are the units it is measuring? If it is a map, what does it depict and what is the map scale?

On the TEAS test, graphics are always accompanied by a problem. Ask yourself, how can I use the graphic to solve the problem?

For graphics problems, you will not be asked to make complicated analyses or calculations. Instead, you will be asked about general trends in the graphic and how they relate to the problem you have to solve.

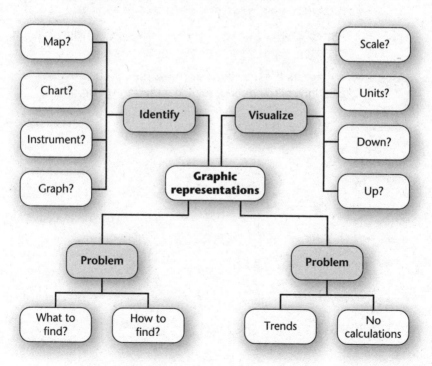

The Reading portion of the TEAS exam may present any of several kinds of graphics. These may include the following:

- A **bar graph** compares data using vertical or horizontal bars to represent numerical values.

- A **line graph** plots data points on a grid and connects them with a line to show trends.

- A **pie chart** shows relative values by dividing a circle into wedges that represent percentages of the whole.

- A **flow chart** shows a procedure or sequence in order by connecting boxes with arrows.

- A **table** compares two or more sets of data in columns or rows.

- A **map** depicts an area, such as a country, city, neighborhood, or factory setup, and its most important features.

- A **diagram** is a drawing that shows the structure or inner workings of something, such as a machine or organism.

R.1.6 PROBLEMS

Use the map to answer the following two questions. Assume you are located at position A on Piermont Drive.

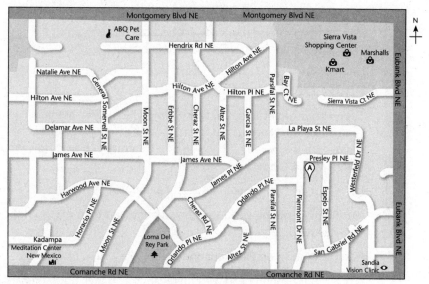

R.1.6 PROBLEM 1

Which of the following identifies the best way to get to Eubank Boulevard from your location on Piermont Drive?

(A) north on Piermont, right on San Gabriel to Eubank

(B) south on Piermont, right on Presley, right on Westerfeld, left on San Gabriel to Eubank

(C) south on Piermont, west on Comanche to Eubank

(D) south on Piermont, left on San Gabriel to Eubank

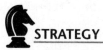 STRATEGY

Follow each route. Find the simplest and best route.

THINK

- Answer choice (A) is incorrect because going north on Piermont will not take you to San Gabriel.

- Answer choice (B) is incorrect because going south on Piermont will not take you to Presley.

- Answer choice (C) is incorrect because going west on Comanche will take you away from Eubank, not toward Eubank.

- Answer choice (D) is correct because it takes you to the intersection of San Gabriel and Eubank.

R.1.6 PROBLEM 2

Suppose you want to get to Montgomery Boulevard but you can't travel on Hendrix Road or across Hendrix Road because the entire road is blocked off because of a water main break. How would you head out to reach Montgomery?

(A) From Piermont, head south to Comanche.

(B) From Piermont, head west on Orlando and then make a right on Harwood.

(C) Head north on Piermont and then make a right on Presley.

(D) From Piermont, head west on Orlando and then north on Parsifal.

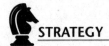 STRATEGY

Follow each route. Find the simplest and best one.

THINK

- Answer choices (B), (C), and (D) all will eventually either be on Hendrix or need to cross Hendrix in order to get to Montgomery.

- That leaves (A) as the only correct response. You would take Comanche east to Eubank and then go north on Eubank until you hit Montgomery.

R.1.7 RECOGNIZE EVENTS IN A SEQUENCE

Recognizing sequence in a text helps the reader recall important points and understand the meaning of the text. Often events or ideas are placed in a logical sequential order to make them easier to grasp.

It is important to remember that sequential order is not exactly the same as chronological order. Chronological order places events in the order in which they happened—strictly in time order. Sequential order can refer to other kinds of fixed order, such as the pages in a book, the house numbers on a street, or the steps in a lab experiment.

On the TEAS Reading exam, you must be able to recognize how events or ideas are presented in a sequence.

- Identify words in the text that signal sequential order, such as *first, next,* and *finally.*

- Note the order of the events or ideas. Look for ways in which they are logically connected.

- Consider what the overall sequence of events or ideas tells you about the topic or main point of the text.

Words that show sequential order include the following:

first	second	third	next
before	initial	next	prior to
after	final	last	then
start	end	finally	ultimately

Words that show chronological order include the following:

now	then	today	yesterday
tomorrow	earlier	later	during
until	when	since	preceding
while	soon	previously	yet

Notice the words that present a logical sequence in this passage.

> **Before** the legislators voted on the bill, they debated its possible effects. **Initially,** passage of the bill seemed unlikely. **Then** an influential member changed her position. This was the breakthrough that **ultimately** won the day.

To recognize a sequence of events, look for words that signal sequential order or chronological order.

R.1.7 PROBLEM

Read the passage. Then answer the question.

Vanessa began to ride her bike every day. Prior to adopting this routine, she rarely got any exercise. Afterward, Vanessa noticed she had more energy and stamina. The next thing she wants to do is join a gym and learn yoga.

Which of the following occurred first in this sequence?

(A) Vanessa noticed she had more energy and stamina.

(B) Vanessa began to ride her bike every day.

(C) Vanessa decided she wants to join a gym and learn yoga.

(D) Vanessa rarely got any exercise.

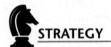 STRATEGY

To answer the question, look for words in the passage that show sequence.

THINK

- The passage contains several words that show sequence, such as *began, prior to, afterward,* and *next.*

- Answer (A) occurred third in sequence, after Vanessa began to ride her bike.

- Answer (B) actually occurred second in sequence, although it is the first sentence in the passage.

- Answer (C) occurred fourth or last in sequence, after Vanessa noticed her gain in energy and stamina from riding her bike.

- Answer (D) occurred first in sequence. Before she began to ride her bike—or prior to adopting this routine—Vanessa rarely got any exercise. Answer (D) is correct.

R.2 CRAFT AND STRUCTURE

R.2.1 DISTINGUISH BETWEEN FACT AND OPINION, BIASES, AND STEREOTYPES

When you read an article or essay, think about the writer's point of view. Does the writer present facts about the topic or personal opinions? On the TEAS Reading exam, you must be able to distinguish between facts and opinions in a text. You should also be able to identify examples of bias or stereotyping.

As you read, examine the writer's point of view and the overall tone of the text.

See whether the writer's statements in the text are mostly facts or opinions. A fact is a statement that can be verified with evidence. An opinion is a statement that reflects a person's personal judgment and may or may not be supported by evidence. Pay attention to the sources the writer cites as evidence.

Look for examples of bias in the text. A bias is a prejudice based on personal beliefs or experience. Bias can be blatantly unfair and irrational, as in racial prejudice. It can also be the product of a person's circumstances, as when, say, a volleyball coach is biased in favor of her team.

Look for examples of stereotypes in the text. A stereotype is an attempt to categorize a person, thing, or idea based on personal prejudice or conventional notions.

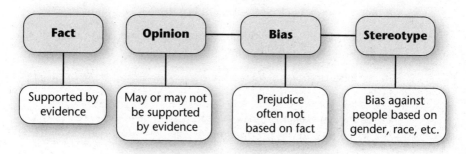

Fact	Opinion	Bias	Stereotype
Supported by evidence	May or may not be supported by evidence	Prejudice often not based on fact	Bias against people based on gender, race, etc.

A person's point of view can affect how he or she approaches a topic. Look at this example:

> In my twenty years in the oil business, I've never seen a more promising development than hydraulic fracturing, or fracking. Fracking is a technique for extracting oil and gas from rock formations deep underground. It is making so-called experts who have long predicted a decline in oil and gas production look extremely foolish. In short, fracking is revolutionizing the energy industry by providing new sources for oil and gas production. Fears about contaminating groundwater and causing earthquakes are based on faulty information. The truth about fracking can be found in my new book on this incredible breakthrough.

Notice that the writer has worked for years in the oil business. This background might affect the writer's point of view in favor of fracking. It is an example of bias that you should look for as you read a text.

To distinguish between fact and opinion in a text, look for statements that are not supported by evidence but merely express a writer's point of view. These can include examples of bias or stereotyping.

You must also distinguish between facts and opinions in the passage. A fact is a verifiable true statement, like the following:

Fact: Fracking is a technique for extracting oil and gas from rock formations deep underground.

In contrast, an opinion includes a person's personal views or beliefs, like the following:

Opinion: It is making so-called experts who have long predicted a decline in oil and gas production look extremely foolish.

Notice that the writer's belief that the experts look foolish is not supported by any evidence.

R.2.1 PROBLEM

Read the passage. Then answer the question.

Law enforcement officials say that texting while driving is a growing problem among teenagers in the United States. According to a poll conducted by the American Automobile Association (AAA), 35% of teen drivers admitted to texting and driving even though they are aware of the dangers. Texting while driving causes one out of every four auto accidents in the United States each year. Most of these accidents are undoubtedly the fault of teenage girls, who seem careless and rarely pay attention while driving. It is important for young drivers in particular to set their phones aside while driving. According to AAA, about eleven teens lose their lives every day because they were texting while driving.

Which of the following sentences from the passage is the writer's opinion?

(A) Law enforcement officials say that texting while driving is a growing problem among teenagers in the United States.

(B) Most of these accidents are undoubtedly the fault of teenage girls, who seem careless and rarely pay attention while driving.

(C) According to a poll conducted by AAA, 35% of teen drivers admitted to texting and driving even though they are aware of the dangers.

(D) According to AAA, about eleven teens lose their lives every day because they were texting while driving.

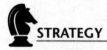 STRATEGY

An opinion includes personal beliefs or biases. An opinion cannot be verified like a fact.

THINK

- Answer (A) provides information from law enforcement officials, so it is a factual statement.

- Answers (C) and (D) are statements verified by polls and statistics from the travel organization AAA.

- Answer (B) is not backed up by any statistics. It expresses the writer's personal opinion and may also be an example of stereotyping. Answer (B) is correct.

R.2.2 RECOGNIZE THE STRUCTURE OF TEXTS IN VARIOUS FORMATS

There are three main modes of writing: persuasive, expository, and narrative. Persuasive writing tries to convince the reader to believe something or presents an argument. Expository writing describes something or presents personal reactions or feelings, as in articles and personal essays. Narrative writing tells a story, as in myths, legends, fables, short stories, novels, and plays. On the TEAS Reading exam, you must recognize these modes of writing, plus various text structures in persuasive and expository writing.

Text structure organizes the material and provides clues to the reader about the meaning of the text. Look for:

- **Sequence as a text structure.** This can take the form of a list, numbered steps, or information organized in outline form. Sequence may also be used to show how something has changed over time or how events unfolded in history.

- **A problem/solution text structure.** This introduces a problem in the first paragraph or section and then provides a solution to the problem in the remainder of the text.

- **A cause/effect text structure.** This describes an event or action in one paragraph and goes on to show the effects or consequences of that event in the following paragraph.

- **A compare/contrast text structure.** This presents similarities and differences between people, places, things, or ideas.

Now, let's look at examples of the main types of text structure.

Sequence: A text describes, decade by decade, how the comic book character Superman has changed from his first appearance in 1938 to today.

Problem and solution: The first paragraph of a text describes a problem with local landfills becoming overfilled. The paragraph that follows describes a recycling program that aims to solve the problem.

Cause and effect: A text describes a tsunami in the first paragraph. The following paragraphs describe the damage done by the tsunami and the effect on the population.

Compare and contrast: A text describes the similarities and differences of two popular cellphone models.

To recognize the structure of texts in various formats, you must know the different methods for organizing a text, such as sequence, cause/effect, compare/contrast, and problem/ solution.

Another text structure that is frequently used in persuasive writing is **claim and evidence**. A writer might claim that all students in high school should receive laptop computers. The writer then might present evidence that using laptop computers improves student performance in several areas. The writer might also anticipate counterclaims to the original idea and provide responses to these objections.

R.2.2 PROBLEM

Read the passage. Then answer the question.

It is annoying to see paper cups and aluminum cans alongside roads and highways. Public parks often have sheets of newspaper and plastic bags blowing across the grounds. There are many ways an individual can help keep litter to a minimum. Always have a litterbag in your vehicle and hang on to your trash until you can throw it in a garbage receptacle. Take a trash bag with you to the park when you cook out with friends. At home, put loose newspapers in a paper sack before putting them in your recycling bin. Work with friends and neighbors to join an adopt-a-road beautification program or go out on weekends to pick up litter in parks and on vacant lots and roadsides.

Which type of text structure does the writer of this passage use?

(A) cause and effect

(C) sequential

(B) problem and solution

(D) compare and contrast

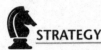

STRATEGY

Remember the most common text structures: **sequence, problem-solution, cause and effect,** and **compare-contrast.**

THINK

- Which text structure fits this passage best?

- The writer describes a problem in the opening sentences of the paragraph—getting rid of litter in public places. Then the writer presents several ways this can be accomplished.

- The writer has raised a problem and offered several possible solutions. Answer (B) is correct.

R.2.3 INTERPRET THE MEANING OF WORDS AND PHRASES USING CONTEXT

To understand a text, readers should have a strategy to figure out the meanings of unfamiliar words and phrases. They must also interpret words with multiple meanings, technical language, and the use of figurative language. On the TEAS Reading exam, you must employ various strategies to show comprehension of words in context.

Look for words that are unfamiliar or have multiple meanings. Use context clues to determine the correct meaning. Context clues are found in the text before and after the word you must define. Sometimes the text contains a definition of the word or an illustration of what it is.

Examine the structure of unfamiliar words to determine their meaning. Think about the meaning of the root word. Notice how the meaning is changed by the word's prefix or suffix.

Identify figurative language such as similes, metaphors, and hyperbole. Authors use figurative language to emphasize important points and reveal their attitude toward the topic.

The context clues surrounding an unfamiliar word provide hints to the word's meaning. Use the following strategies to make informed guesses about a word's meaning.

Look for a **definition** of the word.

> Carnavon then found a large jeweled cup among the treasures and assumed the goblet was the ancient king's **chalice**. (A *chalice* is a large cup or goblet.)

Look for a **synonym** of the word.

> The scientist's purview, or primary field, was limited to molecular biology. (*Purview* is a person's primary field of study or expertise.)

Look for an **antonym** of the word.

> After **chastising** Rex for his poorly written story, Gina felt so bad that she spent the next hour praising his writing skills. (*Chastising* is the opposite of praising; it means "scolding or criticizing.")

Compare or contrast the word with surrounding words or phrases.

> The sauce contained honey, but it was not at all **saccharine**, like the sugar-rich syrup that Hal had poured on the cake. (*Saccharine* means "sickeningly sweet.")

Look at the **context or situation**.

> Paula took a shot at the basket, but the ball missed badly, clanked off the rim, and **caromed** back to Paula. (*Caromed* means "rebounded.")

Replace the unfamiliar word with your guess.

> The room was filled with **opulent** furnishings that were beautiful and clearly expensive. (Replace *opulent* with the word you guess is close to its meaning: *luxurious*. Then see if the sentence makes sense.)

Look at the **root and affixes** of the unfamiliar word.

> No one knew that the ambassador had traveled to the conference and attended several lectures **incognito**. (The root *cognit-* means "to get to know." The prefix *in-* means "not." *Incognito* means "in disguise so as not to be known or recognized.")

Also look for examples of figurative language, like the following.

Simile: The National Gem Collection contains a large uncut emerald that looks **like an enormous chunk of green ice.** (A simile compares two things using *like* or *as.* The emerald is compared to a chunk of green ice.)

Metaphor: The colonel's voice **was a foghorn** in the darkness, calling the men to attention. (A metaphor compares two things without using *like* or *as.* The voice is compared to a foghorn, so it must be deep and loud.)

Hyperbole: We waited at the airport **for an eternity,** but our cousin never arrived. (The word *eternity* conveys that we waited a very long time.)

To interpret the meaning of words and phrases in context, look for word structure, including root words and affixes, and clues in surrounding words and sentences.

R.2.3 PROBLEM

Read the sentence. Then answer the question.

The six-time Grammy winner was walking down the sidewalk in New York City when she was <u>beset</u> by a mass of fans shouting her name.

Which of the following is a synonym for the underlined word in the sentence?

(A) helped

(B) threatened

(C) surrounded

(D) consoled

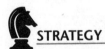

STRATEGY

Remember that a synonym is a word with the same meaning as another word. You can use context clues to figure out which word is a synonym for the underlined word.

THINK

- Refer to the situation in the sentence and use your real-world knowledge to make an intelligent guess about which word is a synonym for the underlined word.

- Notice that a famous person is walking down the street in New York City. The fans are shouting her name.

- They are unlikely to be helping her in this situation, so (A) is incorrect. They are coming toward her rather than resisting her, so (B) is incorrect. It makes no sense for the fans to be consoling the celebrity, so (D) is also incorrect.

- The correct answer is (C). The celebrity is suddenly surrounded by her excited fans.

R.2.4 EVALUATE THE AUTHOR'S PURPOSE IN A GIVEN TEXT

When you read a text, think about what the writer is trying to do. Recognizing the author's purpose will help you comprehend what you read. On the TEAS, you must be able to determine an author's main purpose in a given text.

Ask yourself which of the following the writer is trying to do:

- **Inform the reader about the topic.** An informational text concentrates on facts that can be verified. It may be divided into short sections for easier reading. It may also include special features such as section heads, numbered or bulleted lists, and graphics such as charts, maps, and diagrams. An encyclopedia article, a museum catalog, and a set of instructions are all informational texts.

- **Persuade the reader** to do something or believe some proposition. A persuasive text includes emotional language along with factual material. It may employ bias or propaganda in an attempt to sway the reader.

- **Entertain the reader.** A text that entertains may be a suspenseful novel, a scary short story, a humorous essay, or a nostalgic blog post.

- **Express personal feelings.** An expressive text uses colorful or poetic language to create word pictures and summon strong emotions. It may be in the form of a poem or personal essay.

Here are some examples of texts about dogs, each with a different purpose.

Inform: A description of how different dog breeds are classified.

Persuade: A blog post that tells why beagles are the best breed of dog.

Entertain: An account of how the writer's dog ran off with the Thanksgiving turkey.

Express Feelings: A prose poem that explores the writer's attachment to her dog.

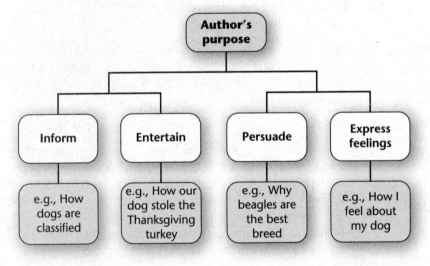

To evaluate the author's purpose in a text, read carefully to decide why it was written. The author might be trying to inform, persuade, entertain, or express personal feelings.

You should also remember that an author may have more than one purpose in writing a text. For example, an article that tries to persuade people to donate to a charity that fights cancer may also express personal feelings about the writer's own experience with cancer. An informative piece on the statistics of cellphone use may be written in a breezy, entertaining style.

R.2.4 PROBLEM

Read the paragraph. Then answer the question.

The numbers regarding computer usage in U.S. public schools are troubling. Statistics show that public schools have fewer computers per student than private schools. Teachers of low-income students are more than twice as likely to see lack of internet access as a major challenge than teachers of high-income students. This so-called digital divide threatens to sabotage educational opportunities for millions of underprivileged young Americans. In today's world of constantly changing digital technology, students must have access to personal computers, laptops, or tablets as a vital part of their education. These devices help students do research, manage course materials, and complete assignments. It is time for the federal government to create a program to provide more computers for schools. This will ensure that our children are learning the technical skills necessary to enter the workforce and find good jobs.

Which of the following is the author's main purpose in this passage?

(A) express personal feelings about the challenges faced by low-income students

(B) persuade the reader to support a federal program to put more computers in American public school classrooms

(C) entertain the reader with an amusing account of how education has changed over the years

(D) inform the reader about statistics of computer availability and usage in U.S. public and private schools

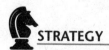 STRATEGY

Authors generally have one of four purposes for writing: to **explain**, to **persuade**, to **entertain**, or to **express feelings**.

THINK

- The author does express personal feelings about the issue of computers in schools, but this is not the main purpose of the passage. Answer (A) is incorrect.

- The passage does not seek to entertain readers with an amusing account of changes in education, so answer (C) is incorrect.

- The passage does begin with some information about computers in public and private schools, but the actual statistics are not provided and this is not the author's main purpose. Answer (D) is incorrect.

- The author does refer to these statistics to support the case for a federal program. The author is trying to persuade the reader that such a program is needed. Answer (B) is correct.

R.2.5 EVALUATE THE AUTHOR'S POINT OF VIEW IN A GIVEN TEXT

In opinion pieces, such as editorials and political endorsements, a writer's point of view is presented straightforwardly. However, point of view can also be found in informational writing. Writers are not machines that produce balanced, factual material at will. Even when writing a news story or fact-based account, a writer often will reveal his or her point of view about the topic. On the TEAS exam, you will examine texts and evaluate the author's point of view about the topic.

- When reading a text, note the author's name and background and the name of the publication in which the text appears. Notice whether the author works for a group that might provide clues about his or her viewpoint.

- As you read, think about the context and purpose of the text. Was it written to persuade the reader about something? Was it written on a special occasion? Does it support its point of view with facts and expert opinions?

- Decide whether you think the author's information is accurate and reliable. Ask yourself if you agree with the author's point of view. Look for signs of personal bias in the text. If the author takes an extreme position on some issue, you might read other pieces on the same topic to compare points of view.

Look at these examples of point of view in a text and think about how each person's point of view might be different.

An op-ed piece about genetically modified crops written by

- the owner of an all-natural farmer's market.

- a salesperson for a company that produces and sells genetically modified seeds.

- a scientist who studies the benefits and possible hazards of genetically modified food.

The owner of the farmer's market would probably favor naturally grown crops over genetically modified versions. The owner's business appeals to people who are opposed to genetically modified crops. The salesperson would probably insist that genetically modified seeds produce plants with certain important advantages, such as resistance to being eaten by insects. The salesperson depends on selling genetically modified seeds for his or her livelihood. The scientist might offer a more balanced point of view about genetically modified crops. The scientist is trained to do research in a rigorous, fair-minded manner. However, it might be important to find out whom the scientist works for.

To evaluate the author's point of view in a given text, read carefully to determine the author's assumptions and biases about the topic. Also think about the source of the text, such as where it was published and who sponsored it.

R.2.5 PROBLEM

Which of the following would be most likely to write an editorial in favor of tougher gun-control laws?

(A) a member of the National Rifle Association

(B) a person who owns a shooting range

(C) a rural homeowner who keeps a rifle in the house for protection from prowlers

(D) a person who believes that legal gun ownership is reserved for police officers or state militias, not private citizens

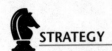

STRATEGY

Think about what point of view a person who favors tougher gun-control laws would probably have.

THINK

- The National Rifle Association member would probably be opposed to tougher gun-control laws as a matter of political belief, so answer (A) is incorrect.

- The owner of a shooting range would probably support more lenient gun-control laws to increase his or her business, so answer (B) is incorrect.

- The rural homeowner would not favor tougher gun-control laws that might take away the right to keep a gun for self-defense. Answer (C) is incorrect.

- The person who believes legal gun ownership is only for police officers or members of state militias would be more likely to favor tougher gun-control laws philosophically. Answer (D) is correct.

R.2.6 USE TEXT FEATURES

Text features are included in a text, but are not components of the main body of text, to help the reader find information or use it more effectively. Informational text such as magazine articles often contains many different text features to make the material look more inviting or to provide related facts. On the TEAS Reading exam, you should demonstrate an understanding of text features and how to use them.

First, look for headings and subheadings in the text. These might be in all capital letters, in larger type, or in boldface. Headings are generally larger than subheadings. Notice how the headings and subheadings divide the material into different sections or subtopics.

Next, look for features that are placed outside the text. These can include sidebars and footnotes. Sidebars are sentences or short paragraphs located at the side of the main text or set off in boxes. They present additional information about the topic. Footnotes are found at the bottom of the page and indicate the original source for quoted material in the text.

Finally, look for special typefaces used to highlight words in the text. Italic type may be used to highlight foreign words or phrases or to emphasize a word, phrase, or sentence. Boldface type is also used for headings and for emphasis.

Other text features found in books include the title page, copyright page, table of contents, photos, illustrations, maps, captions, glossary, and index.

To use text features, be aware of how the text is organized and how certain features such as headings, subheadings, sidebars, footnotes, and italic type are included to make parts of the text easy to find or use.

R.2.6 PROBLEM

Read the text. Then answer the question.

THE 1960 PRESIDENTIAL RACE

A Religious Question

The 1960 presidential election pitted former Republican vice-president Richard M. Nixon against Democratic Senator John F. Kennedy. Foreign policy and Cold War competition with the Soviet Union dominated the race. Yet religion also became an issue in the campaign. Kennedy was Roman Catholic, and some of Nixon's supporters claimed that Kennedy would be loyal to the Pope, not to the U.S. Constitution. Nixon actually instructed his staff *not* to raise the question in the campaign, but the controversy lingered all the way to November.

First Televised Debate

Kennedy and Nixon participated in the first televised presidential debate. The two candidates sparred on the issues of the day, including the economy, the so-called missile gap with Russia, and the new communist regime that had taken power in Cuba. The debate featured strong points on both sides. Oddly, however, the television cameras seemed to decide the outcome. Those who listened to the debate on the radio thought that Nixon won, while those who watched on TV favored Kennedy. Nixon spoke with authority but sweated profusely under the hot lights of the studio, making him look nervous and desperate. Kennedy's suave manner before the camera lens won the day. As historian Theodore H. White wrote, "Every American election summons the individual voter to weigh the past against the future."* Kennedy seemed to represent the future to American voters. In a close election, he won the presidency.

---

* Theodore H. White, *The Making of the President 1960,* Atheneum House, 1961.

What is the main purpose of the footnote in this text?

(A) to explain the topic of the second paragraph

(B) to explain why religion became an issue in the 1960 presidential campaign

(C) to provide the source of the quote in the second paragraph

(D) to provide additional information about the 1960 election

 STRATEGY

Read the footnote in the passage. Remember what a footnote tells the reader.

THINK

- Answer (A) is incorrect because the footnote does not explain the topic of the second paragraph.

- Answer (B) is incorrect because the footnote does not explain why religion became an issue in the campaign.

- Answer (D) is incorrect because, even though the book cited does provide lots of additional information about the campaign, that is not its main purpose in this text.

- The main purpose of the footnote is to give the source of the quote. Answer (C) is correct.

R.3 INTEGRATION OF KNOWLEDGE AND IDEAS

R.3.1 IDENTIFY PRIMARY SOURCES IN VARIOUS MEDIA

Historians value primary sources because they are closest to the people who actually lived during a certain time period or participated in historical events. These sources were created at the time being studied. A statue or piece of pottery is a primary source for studying an ancient civilization. An eyewitness account in a journal, a photograph, an audio recording, or a video are all firsthand sources for studying a modern event. On the TEAS Reading exam, you must evaluate various types of sources to see if they are primary or secondary.

To identify a primary source, think about the author's relationship to the text material or event. If the author participated in the event or was an eyewitness, the source is primary.

Take note of the publication date of the source. If it is not close to the date of the event described, it is probably not a primary source.

Evaluate the purpose of the source. If its main purpose is to provide a factual, firsthand account of an event, it may be considered a primary source.

The following are some examples of primary sources:

- artifacts
- photographs and videos
- artistic works, such as paintings, films, or recordings
- diaries and journals
- letters
- speeches
- memoirs or autobiographies
- interviews
- legal documents
- records of legislative proceedings

To identify primary sources in various media, look for sources that have not been changed, adapted, or interpreted by someone other than the original creator.

Secondary sources analyze an event after it has happened— sometimes long afterward. Secondary sources often make use of primary sources for their analysis. Secondary sources include the following:

- magazine articles

- biographies

- history books

- textbooks

- encyclopedias and reference books

R.3.1 PROBLEM

Which of the following is a primary source about the jazz artist Louis Armstrong?

(A) an interview with a jazz musician who once played with Armstrong

(B) a blog post about how Armstrong revolutionized jazz

(C) an entry from Armstrong's personal journal

(D) a speech about Armstrong's influence on young musicians today

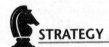 STRATEGY

Remember that in a primary source, the author participated in the events or witnessed them firsthand.

THINK

- A primary source on Louis Armstrong would be in his own words.

- Since the interview is not with Armstrong himself, answer (A) is not correct.

- The blog post and the speech discuss Armstrong, but are not written by him. Answers (B) and (D) are incorrect.

- The entry from Armstrong's personal journal is written in his own words, so it is a primary source. Answer (C) is correct.

R.3.2 USE EVIDENCE FROM TEXT TO MAKE PREDICTIONS AND INFERENCES, AND DRAW CONCLUSIONS ABOUT A PIECE OF WRITING

As a reader, it is enjoyable to figure out what is really happening in a story without being told by the author. Good writers often withhold certain information and leave it up to the reader to figure out what is going on, what the characters' motives are, and what will happen next. The reader gathers clues and details like pieces of a puzzle and fits them together to draw logical conclusions. On the TEAS Reading exam, you must use evidence from a text to make predictions, infer meaning, and draw conclusions.

To make a prediction about a text, use details to deduce something that will occur in the future. Often, an author will insert hints and clues about how the story will develop. This is a technique called foreshadowing.

> **Example:** In a story about an unconventional teacher, the teacher uses computer games to motivate a troubled student who is failing. Based on story details, you might predict that the student will become a computer whiz and earn a scholarship to college. You reason that if the author spends so much time describing this unconventional teaching method, it must be a method that ultimately pays off.

To make an inference (a more subtle form of prediction), use your personal experience and details from the text to "read between the lines" and make assumptions about the story.

> **Example:** A teenager in a story refuses to try for a driver's license despite having a car available at home. The character grows nervous when discussing the matter with friends. You might infer that the character has a phobia about driving. Then you can use active reading techniques to confirm or disprove your inference as you learn more information about the character.

To draw a conclusion, use details from the text to decide what the ending means or what the overall theme is.

> **Example:** In Charles Dickens' *A Christmas Carol,* the reader learns that Ebenezer Scrooge is a miserly curmudgeon who has lost the ability to love and feel pity. Through visits from the Ghosts of Christmas Past, Present, and Future, Scrooge realizes what he has missed by focusing on money not people. You can draw the conclusion that Dickens wants to show that love and charitable feelings are more important than material things.

To make predictions and draw conclusions about a piece of writing, look for significant details that provide clues about what will happen next or how the story will end.

A reader can also make predictions and draw conclusions about other elements of a text. For example, you can predict the meaning of an unfamiliar word from context clues. You can draw conclusions about what kind of text you are reading by noticing special features, such as bulleted lists, sidebars, maps, or graphs.

R.3.2 PROBLEM

Read the passage. Then answer the question.

It wasn't that Marie disliked the new girl at her high school. Lucinda Graham had an easy smile and a humble manner, and she got along well with almost everyone. The problem arose when Lucinda began to outdo Marie at Marie's traditional specialties. For example, Lucinda joined the softball team and within a week had replaced Marie as the leadoff hitter and shortstop. In the Chess Club, Lucinda forced Marie to resign three times in a row—the first games Marie had ever lost at school! Now there was talk that Lucinda's science project would be chosen as the school's lone entry in the statewide Science Fair, the same fair at which Marie had earned top honors last year. Well, the election for class president was coming up in a month. At least Marie, as the popular incumbent, had that to fall back on.

Which of the following predictions would you make about this story?

(A) Marie will decide not to run for class president.

(B) Lucinda will challenge Marie in the election for class president.

(C) Marie and Lucinda will work together to help someone else become class president.

(D) Lucinda will boast about her victories over Marie and lose popularity among the students.

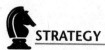

STRATEGY

To make a prediction, use details from the text to figure out what will probably happen in the future.

THINK

- Refer to details from the story to decide which is the most logical prediction.

- You know that answer (A) is incorrect because Marie is looking forward to running for reelection as class president.

- Answer (C) is incorrect because there is no evidence that Marie and Lucinda want to work together in the election.

- Answer (D) is incorrect because Lucinda is not described as boastful but as having a humble manner.

- You can predict that Lucinda will challenge Marie for class president because Lucinda has done this in several other activities. Answer (B) is correct.

R.3.3 COMPARE AND CONTRAST THEMES FROM PRINT AND OTHER SOURCES

The theme of a literary work is the underlying concern or wider message that an author explores. Themes are considered universal because they exist throughout history and across cultures. For example, the theme of coming of age is found in Shakespeare's *Henry IV, Part 1,* Stephen Crane's *The Red Badge of Courage,* and Madeleine L'Engle's *A Wrinkle in Time.* On the TEAS Reading exam, you will compare and contrast themes in literature, nonfiction writing, and other sources.

To find the theme of a text, look for the major idea that the author is addressing. This is not simply the topic of the text, but rather the larger idea that underlies the story. For example, a detective story set in a large city may deal with the overall theme of corruption in high places.

To compare how two authors approach a similar theme, think about the underlying message each author delivers about the theme. Remember that a classic theme such as romantic jealousy can be treated in different ways. Shakespeare's *Othello* presents the theme of mistaken jealousy as a towering tragedy, while a novelist may present a comic character who becomes jealous because of a silly misunderstanding.

Bear in mind that similar themes can be employed in different genres, such as novels, short stories, film, drama, poetry, and painting. For example, the theme of loneliness is found in George Eliot's novel *Silas Marner*, Martin Scorsese's film *Taxi Driver*, and Edward Hopper's painting *Nighthawks*. You should be able to examine how the theme is addressed in each type of work.

To compare and contrast themes from print and other sources, think about the wider universal concepts that authors mean to address in stories, essays, or articles.

Some common themes that are found in many works across many time periods and cultures include the following:

- Betrayal
- Change versus tradition
- Community
- Disillusionment with life
- Fading beauty
- Family
- Friendship
- Heroism
- Homecoming
- Individual versus society
- Injustice
- Loss of innocence
- Love
- Motherhood
- Nature and beauty
- Power and corruption
- Racial prejudice
- Rebirth
- Self-reliance
- Temptation
- Tragedy of war
- Vanity

R.3.3 PROBLEM

Read the passage. Then answer the question.

In Ernest Hemingway's short novel *The Old Man and the Sea,* an old Cuban fisherman has gone eighty-four days without catching a fish, although he keeps trying day after day. He is mocked by the other fishermen for his failures. The parents of his young apprentice forbid the boy to accompany the old man any longer because he is deemed unlucky. Finally, on the eighty-fifth day, the old man hooks a huge marlin and reels in the fish after an exhausting struggle lasting two days. He lashes the marlin to his boat and heads home. However, sharks swarm his little boat and devour the marlin, leaving only its skeleton. The old man manages to get his boat ashore and staggers off to finally get some sleep. The next day a number of fishermen are amazed to see the marlin's eighteen-foot skeleton attached to the boat. They realize the old man has made an enormous effort to catch the fish and bring it in. The old man's young apprentice promises to accompany him on his next outing.

Which of the following best states the theme of this story?

(A) hopelessness of old age

(B) the difficulty of fishing for marlin

(C) youth versus age

(D) persistence and courage

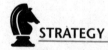 STRATEGY

To find the theme of a story, look for a larger idea that the author is trying to express.

THINK

- Test each answer choice to see if it fits as the overall theme of the passage.

- Even though the protagonist is old, his situation is not hopeless because he keeps trying to succeed. Answer (A) is not correct.

- The difficulty of fishing for marlin is an important element of the story, but it is not the overall theme. Answer (B) is not correct.

- Youth versus age is not the theme, because the apprentice is not competing with the old man. Answer (C) is not correct.

- The old man does show persistence and courage in catching the marlin, even though the sharks spoil his catch. Persistence and courage serves as the overall theme. Answer (D) is correct.

R.3.4 EVALUATE AN ARGUMENT AND ITS SPECIFIC CLAIMS

In a persuasive text, an author will present an argument and try to support it with reasons or evidence. The argument may be presented as something the author believes or favors. It may be preceded by the words "I believe" or "in my opinion." An argument may also be offered as a fact that everyone already believes or accepts. The author then will offer evidence to support his or her argument. On the TEAS Reading exam, you must be able to evaluate an author's argument and the specific claims it makes.

First, identify the author's argument, or the claim he or she is making. Usually this is found early in the text, but it may be stated most clearly at the end.

Next, identify the evidence the author presents to support the argument. These are facts or specific claims provided to convince the reader.

Check the sources for the evidence they provide. The best evidence includes sources that are up to date, clearly stated, unbiased, and peer reviewed or drawn from respected publications. Decide whether the evidence is sufficient to justify the author's claim.

Check for claims that are exaggerated, poorly sourced, or beside the point. If the author does not have good supporting evidence, you may conclude that the argument is weak or flawed.

REMEMBER

To evaluate an author's argument, identify the claim being made and then determine how valid the supporting evidence is.

For example, in an editorial an author might argue that states should spend more to subsidize wind turbines as a clean, efficient source of energy. An article from *Scientific American* that discusses how today's wind turbines are more efficient than ever before would be an excellent piece of evidence to support the author's argument. A quote from the owner of a wind power company would be less convincing because it might be biased. An explanation of how windmills operated in the nineteenth century would be a poor piece of evidence because it is irrelevant to the argument.

The ability to evaluate an argument enables you to read editorials and opinion pieces with a more discerning eye and stay informed about important current issues.

R.3.4 PROBLEM

Read the author's argument. Then answer the question.

The time has come to allow female marathon runners to compete alongside male runners in international competition.

Which of the following claims does not support the argument above?

(A) According to statistics from around the country, more women are entering weekend 5K and 10K races than ever before.

(B) According to *Runner's World* magazine, winning times for women in major marathons worldwide are coming down faster than winning times for men.

(C) A current expert in sports medicine notes that running is a sport that relies on endurance rather than raw strength or speed, so it may be better suited for women to compete with men.

(D) In an interview this year, a major international running coach said that with proper training women could soon become competitive with men in marathons and other distance races.

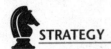

STRATEGY

Compare the supporting details to the author's argument to see if they provide valid support for his or her position.

THINK

- Remember that you are looking for the claim that does NOT support the author's argument.

- Answers (B), (C), and (D) all present valid claims from good sources that support the author's argument.

- Notice that an increase in competitive running among females is not by itself a reason to support the author's argument. Answer (A) is correct.

R.3.5 EVALUATE AND INTEGRATE DATA FROM MULTIPLE SOURCES ACROSS VARIOUS FORMATS

When you are researching a topic, you should seek information from several different sources. Often the data you want is found in graphics, such as charts, graphs, tables, and diagrams. Comparing and contrasting data from different sources helps you comprehend the topic better and draw meaningful conclusions. On the TEAS Reading exam, you must be able to evaluate and integrate data from multiple sources and in a variety of formats.

- Identify the topic for research. Think about what sources of information would be most useful for researching this topic.

- Look up sources and evaluate each one for its usefulness and relevance.

- Compile data from multiple sources and in various formats, such as charts, graphs, tables, and diagrams. Organize the data according to your research needs. Analyze and synthesize the data in order to draw conclusions about your topic.

For example, as a nursing student you might research a new blood-thinning medication. You might seek sources of information about its effectiveness in trials and the risks and side effects involved. A table might compare data about the medication with data for competitors' versions. You can code each piece of data or information to indicate what it tells about the medication and to help you organize it later. For example, data associated with bleeding risks can be coded BR. You might consult with a research librarian or media assistant to find more data from medical journals, online publications, or other approved sources. Once you have compiled all this data, you can analyze it carefully. Your research will enable you to draw meaningful conclusions about the new medication.

To evaluate and integrate data from multiple sources, find data that is most relevant to the topic and organize it in a logical way.

R.3.5 PROBLEM 1

Use the graph to answer the following two questions.

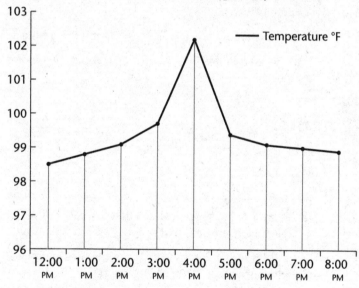

At what time did the patient's temperature spike?

(A) after 2 PM

(C) after 4 PM

(B) after 3 PM

(D) after 5 PM

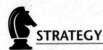

STRATEGY

Read the graph and look for the point that indicates a spike, or sudden rise, in temperature.

THINK

- The temperature spike occurs when the graph rises most steeply.
- The steepest rise on the graph occurs just after 3 PM. This makes answer (B) the correct response.

R.3.5 PROBLEM 2

You are examining a case in which a nurse gave a patient acetaminophen at 3:20 PM. According to the graph, how long did the patient's temperature continue to rise after the acetaminophen was administered?

(A) about 1 hour

(C) about 1.5 hours

(B) about 20 minutes

(D) about 40 minutes

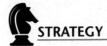

STRATEGY

Read the graph and interpret the data.

THINK

- From the graph, you can tell that the patient's temperature reached its maximum at 4 PM.
- 4 PM is forty minutes from when the medication was administered at 3:20 PM. Answer (D) is correct.

MATHEMATICS

The second section of the TEAS covers Mathematics. It features 34 scored items. There are two categories of Mathematics objectives for the TEAS. The test items are divided among the Mathematics objectives as follows.

M.1 NUMBERS AND ALGEBRA—16 SCORED QUESTIONS

M.1.1   Convert among non-negative fractions, decimals, and percentages.

M.1.2   Perform arithmetic operations with rational numbers.

M.1.3   Compare and order rational numbers.

M.1.4   Solve equations in one variable.

M.1.5   Solve real-world problems using operations with rational numbers.

M.1.6   Solve real-world problems involving percentages.

M.1.7   Apply estimation strategies and rounding rules to real-world problems.

M.1.8   Solve real-world problems involving proportions.

M.1.9   Solve real-world problems involving ratios and rates of change.

M.1.10 Translate phrases and sentences into expressions, equations, and inequalities.

M.2 MEASUREMENT AND DATA—18 SCORED QUESTIONS

M.2.1   Interpret relevant information from tables, charts, and graphs.

M.2.2   Evaluate the information in data sets, tables, charts, and graphs using statistics.

M.2.3   Explain the relationship between two variables.

M.2.4   Calculate geometric quantities.

M.2.5   Convert within and between standard and metric systems.

In addition, the TEAS Mathematics section features four unscored items (aka "pretest" items). These items can address objectives from any of the above categories. You will have 57 minutes to complete the entire Mathematics section.

M.1 NUMBERS AND ALGEBRA

M.1.1 CONVERT AMONG NON-NEGATIVE FRACTIONS, DECIMALS, AND PERCENTAGES

Numerical values are expressed in many different forms, including as fractions, decimals, and percentages. On the Mathematics section of the TEAS exam, you must show that you understand each of these forms and how to convert from one to another.

A **fraction** expresses a ratio, written in the form $\frac{a}{b}$, where a and b are integers. The two parts of a fraction are the numerator and the denominator.

$$\text{fraction} = \frac{\text{numerator}}{\text{denominator}}$$

The value of a fraction is found by dividing the top number (the numerator) by the bottom number (the denominator). A fraction also tells how many parts of a whole there are. For example, the fraction $\frac{3}{4}$ means three parts of a whole with four total parts.

A **decimal** is a number expressed in **place values** based on powers of 10. This is called **decimal notation**.

Decimal notation includes the **decimal point**. Digits to the left of the decimal point show values greater than one. Digits to the right of the decimal point show values less than one.

Look at the chart of place value below. The value of a digit in a number depends on its position, or place value. The chart shows place values for the number 24,628,341.789. Notice that the decimal point separates the ones place from the tenths place.

ten millions	millions	hundred thousands	ten thousands	thousands	hundreds	tens	ones	tenths	hundredths	thousandths
2	4,	6	2	8,	3	4	1.	7	8	9

This number can be read as twenty-four million, six hundred twenty-eight thousand, three hundred forty-one and seven hundred eighty-nine thousandths. Notice that the decimal point is read as "and."

The place value of a decimal tells what the fractional denominator will be.

tens	units	decimal point	tenths	hundredths	thousandths	ten thousandths
0	0	.	6	7	8	

Here, the last digit of the decimal is in the thousandths place. So the fractional equivalent is $\frac{678}{1000}$, or 678 thousandths.

To keep the digits in a decimal in the correct place, fill in zeros. For example, 8 thousandths is written as 0.008, with the 8 in the third place to the right of the decimal point.

If the decimal point is moved to the right, the value of the decimal is increased by a factor of 10. For example, if the decimal point in 0.062 is moved one place to the right, the result is 0.62, which is 10 times larger than the original decimal. Moving the decimal point 2 places to the right multiplies the original decimal by 100, 3 places multiplies by 1,000, and so on.

If the decimal point is moved to the left, the value of the decimal is decreased by a factor of 10. For example, if the decimal point in 0.35 is moved one place to the left, the result is 0.035, which is 10 times smaller than the original decimal. Moving the decimal point 2 places to the left divides the original decimal by 100, 3 places by 1,000, and so on.

A **percentage**, or **percent**, is a special ratio that compares a quantity to 100. For example, 5% means "5 out of 100," 37% means "37 out of 100," and 62.5% means "62.5 out of 100."

To convert among non-negative fractions, decimals, and percentages, remember how the numerator relates to the denominator in a fraction; review place value within decimals; and be able to express a percentage as a numerical part of one hundred.

Fractions, decimals, and percentages all express ratios. The chart below shows how a number of ratios are expressed in these other forms.

Ratio	Fraction	Decimal	Percent
1 out of 100	$\frac{1}{100}$	0.01	1%
5 out of 100	$\frac{1}{20}$	0.05	5%
10 out of 100	$\frac{1}{10}$	0.1	10%
20 out of 100	$\frac{1}{5}$	0.2	20%
33.3 out of 100	$\frac{1}{3}$	0.33	33.3%
25 out of 100	$\frac{1}{4}$	0.25	25%
50 out of 100	$\frac{1}{2}$	0.5	50%
66.7 out of 100	$\frac{2}{3}$	0.67	66.7%
75 out of 100	$\frac{3}{4}$	0.75	75%
90 out of 100	$\frac{9}{10}$	0.9	90%
100 out of 100	1	1.00	100%

Percent to decimal ➞ ÷ 100

Decimal to percent ➞ × 100

For the TEAS Mathematics section, you must be able to convert among fractions, decimals, and percentages.

Converting a fraction to a decimal is done most easily on a calculator. For example, to find the decimal value of $\frac{5}{8}$, divide the numerator 5 by the denominator 8 to get 0.625.

To convert a decimal to a fraction, consider two main situations—when the value is less than 1 and when the value is greater than 1.

- **Less than 1:** Convert 0.84 to a fraction.

  First, write 0.84 divided by 1: $\frac{0.84}{1}$.

  Next, multiply both numerator and denominator by 100 to make the numerator a whole number. (The decimal point must be moved two places to the right.) This gives you $\frac{84}{100}$.

  Finally, simplify the fraction by dividing top and bottom by 4: $\frac{21}{25}$.

- **Greater than 1:** Convert 3.42 to a fraction.

  First, move the decimal point to the right to create a whole number: 342. This is the numerator.

  Next, express the denominator as 1 plus the number of zeros equal to the number of places you moved the decimal point: 100.

  The fraction form of 3.42 is $\frac{342}{100}$. This can be reduced to $\frac{171}{50}$.

To convert a fraction to a percentage, first divide the numerator by the denominator. Then multiply the resulting value by 100 to get the percentage.

$\frac{42}{76} = 0.553 \times 100 = 55.3 = 55.3\%$, which can be rounded to 55%.

To convert a decimal to a percentage, multiply the decimal by 100 by moving the decimal point two places to the right. For example, 0.64 converts to 64%.

M.1.1 PROBLEM 1

How do you write the fraction $40\frac{31}{10,000}$ as a decimal?

(A) 40.31

(C) 40.0031

(B) 40.031

(D) 40.00031

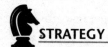

STRATEGY

Use a place value frame.

THINK

- The denominator is 10,000, so write the 1 in the ten thousandths place.

- Write a 3 to the left of the 1.

- Fill in the tens and ones places with 4 and 0, respectively.

hundreds	tens	ones		tenths	hundredths	thousandths	10 thousandths	100 thousandths
	4	0	.	0	0	3	1	

- The tenths and hundredths have no digit, so fill them in with zeros. So $40\frac{31}{10,000} = 40.0031$. The correct response is (C).

M.1.1 PROBLEM 2

How do you write the decimal number 0.016 as a fraction?

(A) $\frac{16}{100}$

(C) $\frac{16}{1,000}$

(B) $\frac{1.6}{1,000}$

(D) $\frac{3}{80}$

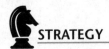

STRATEGY

Place value tells you how to write the fraction.

THINK

- The digit farthest to the right in the decimal tells you the place value.

- The 6 is in the thousandths place. So the denominator of the fraction should be 1,000.

- Write the numerator of 16 into the fraction, giving you $\frac{16}{1,000}$, answer choice (C).

hundreds	tens	ones		tenths	hundredths	thousandths	10 thousandths	100 thousandths
0	0	.		0	1	6		

$\Rightarrow \dfrac{16}{1,000}$

M.1.1 PROBLEM 3

What is the decimal value of 3.5%?

(A) 0.35

(B) 3.5

(C) 0.035

(D) 0.0035

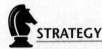

STRATEGY

Use the special "out of 100" ratio of percentages.

THINK

- For this problem, you are going from 3.5% to a decimal, so divide by 100.

- 3.5 ÷ 100 = .035, answer choice (C).

M.1.2 PERFORM ARITHMETIC OPERATIONS WITH RATIONAL NUMBERS

Performing basic calculations by hand is a necessary skill for nurses and allied health professionals, even with a calculator readily available. On the TEAS exam, you must demonstrate the ability to complete computations with the four basic operations on integers, decimals, fractions, and mixed numbers. You also must follow the order of operations when simplifying a mathematical expression.

The four basic mathematical operations are **addition**, **subtraction**, **multiplication**, and **division**.

Basic Operations with Integers

Below are the basic **number facts** for **addition and subtraction**. To use the table, find the intersection of a row and column. For example, 7 + 6 = 13 is shown below.

Addition/Subtraction								
1	**2**	**3**	**4**	**5**	**6**	**7**	**8**	**9**
1	2	3	4	5	6	7	8	9	10
2	3	4	5	6	7	8	9	10	11
3	4	5	6	7	8	9	10	11	12
4	5	6	7	8	9	10	11	12	13
5	6	7	8	9	10	11	12	13	14
6	7	8	9	10	11	12	13	14	15
7	8	9	10	11	12	13	14	15	16
8	9	10	11	12	13	14	15	16	17
9	10	11	12	13	14	15	16	17	18

An excellent learning method for number facts is to create individual flashcards and to drill with them for a few minutes each day.

FLASHCARDS

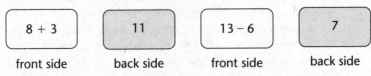

| front side | back side | front side | back side |

Note that knowing an addition fact means that you also know the corresponding subtraction fact by thinking "backward." For example, if you know 3 + 6 = 9, you also know

$$6 + 3 = 9 \rightarrow 9 - 6 = 3 \rightarrow 9 - 3 = 6$$

Similarly, because 7 + 4 = 11:

$$4 + 7 = 11 \rightarrow 11 - 7 = 4 \rightarrow 11 - 4 = 7$$

For numbers with more than one digit, addition and subtraction are done column by column. For example, for 17 + 32,

	1	7
+	3	2
	4	9

If any column adds to more than 9, the value of the tens column in the answer is carried over to the next column to the left. For example, for 27 + 45,

	¹2	7
+	4	5
	7	2

Similarly, if a larger digit is being subtracted from a smaller digit in any column, you have to "borrow" from the column to the left. For example, for 63 – 38, the 3 borrows 10 from the 6. The 3 becomes 13, and the 6 becomes 5 as shown below.

	⁵6	¹3
–	3	8
	2	5

To perform arithmetic operations with rational numbers, you should be able to do computations using the four basic operations with integers, decimals, fractions, and mixed numbers. You should also know and follow the order of operations.

The relationship between addition and subtraction works as a check on any sum or difference that you have calculated.

For example, does 90 − 34 = 56? **Check:** 34 + 56 = 90

Because the sum of 34 and 56 is 90, the answer checks.

In the same way, to check 74 − 45 = 29, add 45 + 29 to see whether the sum is 74. It is, so the answer checks.

The number facts for **multiplication and division** are just as essential as the addition and subtraction facts. Again, to use the table, find the intersection of a row and column. For example, find 7 × 4 = 28.

Multiplication/Division									
	1	2	3	4	5	6	7	8	9
1	1	2	3	4	5	6	7	8	9
2	2	4	6	8	10	12	14	16	18
3	3	6	9	12	15	18	21	24	27
4	4	8	12	16	20	24	28	32	36
5	5	10	15	20	25	30	35	40	45
6	6	12	18	24	30	36	42	48	54
7	7	14	21	28	35	42	49	56	63
8	8	16	24	32	40	48	56	64	72
9	9	18	27	36	45	54	63	72	81

Take some time to make flashcards if you don't know these facts.

FLASHCARDS

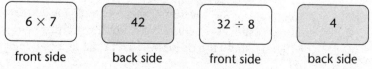

6 × 7	42	32 ÷ 8	4
front side	back side	front side	back side

The backward relationship works for multiplication and division just as it does for addition and subtraction. For example, if you know $8 \times 7 = 56$, you also know

$$7 \times 8 = 56 \rightarrow 56 \div 7 = 8 \rightarrow 56 \div 8 = 7$$

To use the table for division to find, for example, $32 \div 4$, find the first number, 32, in the body of the table, and then find the number to be divided into it in either the top row or left-hand column. Follow the intersection to find the answer. So $32 \div 4 = 8$.

For numbers with more than one digit, multiplication is done by aligning the columns by place value. For example, for 143×2,

1	4	3
	×	2
2	8	6

If any two numbers multiply to more than 9, the value of the tens column in the answer is carried over to the next column to the left, to be added to the next multiplication. Multiply first by the ones column and align that number; then multiply by the tens column and align that number with the tens column, and so on.

For example, for 36×17, the first multiplication is $7 \times 6 \ (= 42)$, so the 2 is placed in the ones column and the 4 carries over for when 7 is multiplied by 3. This gives $(21 + 4) = 25$, so the first multiplication is $7 \times 36 = 252$.

Then for the second multiplication, $1 \times 36 = 36$. That answer is aligned under the 1 (not the 7) because that is the number that was used in the second multiplication. Now add the two results. (Note that a 1 has to be carried over to the left column when 5 and 6 are added.)

		4	
		3	6
		1	7
	1		
	2	5	2
+	3	6	
	6	1	2

Division for numbers with more than one digit is done by setting up the problem as described here. Put the number being divided (**dividend**) under the division sign. Put the number doing the dividing (**divisor**) to the left of the sign. For example, 832 ÷ 16 is set up for long division as follows.

$$16\overline{)832}$$

Divide the divisor (16) into the first digit of the dividend (8). 16 doesn't go into 8, so include the next digit. 16 does go into 83; it goes 5 times (although there will be something left over). So the first number of the answer (**quotient**) is a 5. Be sure to align the 5 over the 3, not the 8, as it is the quotient of 83, not 8. So you have

$$\begin{array}{r} 5 \\ 16\overline{)832} \end{array}$$

Now multiply the quotient by the divisor (5 × 16 = 80) and place this under the 83. Subtract and bring down the next digit (2). The calculation now looks like this:

$$\begin{array}{r} 5 \\ 16\overline{)832} \\ \underline{80} \\ 32 \end{array}$$

Divide the 16 into 32, which goes 2 times. The 2 goes in the quotient above the 2 in the dividend. When the 2 in the quotient is multiplied by the divisor, the answer is 32. The final long division looks like this:

$$\begin{array}{r} 52 \\ 16\overline{)832} \\ \underline{80} \\ 32 \\ \underline{32} \\ 0 \end{array}$$

You can check if the answer is correct by multiplying the quotient 52 by the divisor 16. Indeed, 52 × 16 = 832.

Basic Operations with Fractions

When **adding and subtracting fractions**, you need the fractions to have the same denominator. If the denominators are the same for the fractions, simply add or subtract the numerators and keep the same denominator. Simplify the answer if necessary.

If the denominators of the fractions are different, use the **least common multiple (LCM)** to find the **least common denominator** and convert each fraction to an equivalent fraction with this denominator. For example, if you are adding the fractions $\frac{1}{8}$ and $\frac{1}{6}$, you first must find the LCM of 8 and 6, which is 24. Then you can convert $\frac{1}{8}$ to $\frac{3}{24}$ and $\frac{1}{6}$ to $\frac{4}{24}$. Finally, you have $\frac{3}{24} + \frac{4}{24} = \frac{7}{24}$.

You can also add and subtract **mixed numbers**. A mixed number includes a whole number and a fraction, like $5\frac{3}{5}$. If a problem involves mixed numbers, add or subtract the whole numbers first and then the fractions (as shown above). Then combine the two results. Simplify the answer if necessary.

Multiplying and dividing fractions is actually easier than adding and subtracting them because the fractions can have different denominators.

To multiply fractions, first multiply the numerators to get the numerator of the answer. Then multiply the denominators to get the denominator of the answer. Simplify the answer if necessary. For example,

$$\frac{5}{6} \times \frac{3}{5} = \frac{15}{30} = \frac{1}{2}$$

To multiply mixed numbers, convert them to improper fractions first. An **improper fraction** has a numerator that is larger than its denominator. For example,

$$\frac{5}{6} \times 2\frac{1}{2} = \frac{5}{6} \times \frac{5}{2} = \frac{25}{12} = 2\frac{1}{12}$$

Multiplying fractions can be made easier by **canceling**. If any numerator has a common factor with any denominator, you can divide each by that factor, which simplifies the math at the end. For example, by canceling 4 out of $\frac{5}{8} \times \frac{4}{3}$, you get $\frac{5}{2} \times \frac{1}{3}$, which results in the answer of $\frac{5}{6}$.

To divide fractions, you can "invert and multiply," which means finding the reciprocal of the second fraction and then multiplying as shown above. A **reciprocal** of a fraction is the fraction "flipped over" — with the numerator and denominator swapped. The reciprocal of $\frac{3}{4}$ is $\frac{4}{3}$, and the reciprocal of $\frac{1}{8}$ is 8. Here is an example of invert and multiply:

$$\frac{5}{8} \div \frac{3}{4} = \frac{5}{8} \times \frac{4}{3} = \frac{20}{24} \text{ or } \frac{5}{6}$$

Basic Operations with Decimals

When **adding and subtracting decimals**, be sure to align the decimal points. Fill in zeros if necessary to keep the digits in a decimal in the correct place. Then add or subtract as you usually would.

When multiplying and dividing decimals, you *do not* have to align the decimal points.

Multiply decimals as though the factors were whole numbers, but keep the decimal points where they are. Then follow this procedure to put the decimal point in the correct place in the product.

- Count the total number of digits to the right of the decimal point in both factors.

- Count back to the left from the last digit in the product that same number of places. Place the decimal point there.

- Fill in zeros as necessary.

Divide decimals as though the factors were whole numbers, but keep the decimal points where they are. Follow this procedure to put the decimal point in the correct place in the quotient.

- Count the total number of digits to the right of the decimal point in the divisor.

- Count over this many digits to the right from the decimal point in the dividend.

- Place the decimal point in the quotient at this point.

- Fill in zeros as necessary.

Order of Operations

Order of operations tells you the order in which to simplify a complex expression. The simplest way to remember order of operations is the acronym PEMDAS:

P: Perform calculations inside **p**arentheses

E: Simplify **e**xponents

MD: **M**ultiply and **d**ivide, left to right, before you

AS: **A**dd and **s**ubtract, left to right.

This acronym can also be remembered as **P**lease **E**xcuse **M**y **D**ear **A**unt **S**ally. (Exponents are powers—raised numbers as shorthand to tell how many times a number or variable is a factor of itself. Exponents are not covered on the TEAS exam.)

Here is an example of using order of operations.

$$(12 - 5) \times 4 = \mathbf{(12 - 5)} \times 4 \quad \text{First, perform operations in parentheses.}$$

$$= \mathbf{7 \times 4} \qquad \text{Next, multiply.}$$

$$= 28$$

M.1.2 PROBLEM 1

Find the quotient: $\dfrac{7}{36} \div \dfrac{28}{45}$.

(A) $\dfrac{1}{5}$ (C) $\dfrac{5}{16}$

(B) $\dfrac{3}{4}$ (D) $\dfrac{6}{8}$

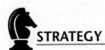 **STRATEGY**

To divide fractions, invert the **divisor** (the number you are dividing by) and multiply.

THINK

- Invert the divisor; then multiply the fractions.

- Cancel factors, as in multiplication.

- After multiplying, check your answer to make sure that it is in lowest terms.

- The correct response is (C).

$$\frac{7}{36} \div \frac{28}{45} =$$

divisor

inverted

$$\frac{{}^{1}\cancel{7}}{\cancel{36}_{4}} \times \frac{{}^{5}\cancel{45}}{\cancel{28}_{4}} = \frac{5}{16}$$

M.1.2 PROBLEM 2

Find the correct answer to this expression: $4 + (18 \div 3) \times 2 = ?$

(A) 14

(C) 20

(B) 16

(D) 48

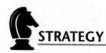

STRATEGY

To find the correct answer, use order of operations.

THINK

- $4 + (18 \div 3) \times 2 = 4 + (18 \div 3) \times 2$ First, perform operations in parentheses.

$$= 4 + 6 \times 2$$ Then multiply.

$$= 4 + 12$$ Then add.

$$= 16$$

- Answer (B) is correct.

M.1.2 PROBLEM 3

Find the sum: $\dfrac{3}{8} + \dfrac{3}{4}$.

(A) $\dfrac{3}{12}$ (C) $\dfrac{6}{16}$

(B) $\dfrac{9}{32}$ (D) $\dfrac{9}{8}$

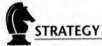 STRATEGY

Use lowest common multiple to find the sum.

THINK

- To find the sum, first find the LCM of 8 and 4, which is 16.
- Convert both fractions to equivalent fractions with the denominator 16. Then add the numerators and simplify.

$$\frac{3}{8} + \frac{3}{4} = \frac{6}{16} + \frac{12}{16} = \frac{18}{16} \text{ or } \frac{9}{8}$$

- Answer choice (D) is correct.

M.1.3 COMPARE AND ORDER RATIONAL NUMBERS

A rational number is any number that can be expressed in fraction form, including decimals, percents, and mixed numbers. You can compare rational numbers using inequality symbols and put them in the correct numeric order. On the TEAS Mathematics exam, you must compare and order rational numbers using the correct terms and symbols.

To compare the numeric values of rational numbers, you must use signs or symbols. These ranking signs include:

     <   less than
     >   greater than
     =   equal to
     ≠   not equal to

≤   less than or equal to

≥   greater than or equal to

These signs (except for the equal sign) are also called **inequality symbols**.

Numeric values can be compared on a **number line**. Values to the left on a number line get smaller. Values to the right get larger.

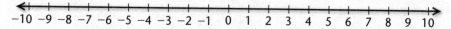

Negative integers are values to the left of 0 on a number line. All negative integers are less than any positive integer. Notice that these negative numbers appear to get larger as you move to the left, from −4 to −5, for example. However, because "negative" can be interpreted as "less than," the values actually do get smaller to the left on the number line. So even though 5 is greater than 3, −5 is less than −3.

To compare the values of fractions, first look at the denominators. If two fractions have the same denominator, compare them by comparing the numerators. For example,

$$\frac{1}{4} < \frac{3}{4} \qquad \frac{5}{8} > \frac{3}{8}$$

Fractions that have different denominators are more difficult to compare. Use the LCD (least common denominator) to convert them to fractions with the same denominator. For example, to find whether $\frac{5}{8}$ is greater or less than $\frac{7}{10}$, find the LCD by finding the lowest common multiple of 8 and 10:

8: 8, 16, 24, 32, **40**, . . .

10: 10, 20, 30, **40**, . . .

So multiply the numerators and denominators of each fraction by a number that will make the denominator 40, which is the LCD.

$$\frac{5}{8} = \frac{5 \times 5}{8 \times 5} = \frac{25}{40} \text{ and } \frac{7}{10} = \frac{7 \times 4}{10 \times 4} = \frac{28}{40}$$

Then, compare the equivalent fractions.

$$\frac{25}{40} < \frac{28}{40} \text{ so } \frac{5}{8} < \frac{7}{10}$$

REMEMBER

To compare and order rational numbers, you must know the symbols for comparing rational numbers or putting them in numeric order from least to greatest and from greatest to least.

Any positive fraction is greater than any negative fraction. For example,

$$\frac{1}{10} > -\frac{9}{10}$$

To compare and order numbers in decimal form, use place value. You can stack the numbers 7.143, 0.756, and 7.046 to compare them by place value.

7.143

0.756

7.046

Comparing them this way, you can order them from least to greatest:

0.756 < 7.046 < 7.143

Where does the fraction $\frac{7}{8}$ fit in this order? Divide 7 by 8 to get a decimal: 0.875. Then place the decimal where it belongs in the inequality.

0.756 < 0.875 < 7.046 < 7.143

Note that the decimals can also be ordered from greatest to least:

7.143 > 7.046 > 0.875 > 0.756

M.1.3 PROBLEM 1

Which of the following numbers has the greatest value?

(A) –7

(B) –2.1

(C) 0

(D) –0.8

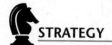

STRATEGY

When ranking or ordering **integers** and **negative numbers**, think of a number line.

THINK

- Here are the four numbers from the series above on the number line.

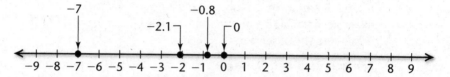

- You can see that 0 is farthest to the right on the number line. So 0 has the greatest value. Answer (C) is correct.

M.1.4 SOLVE EQUATIONS IN ONE VARIABLE

An algebraic equation is a mathematical expression that contains one or more variables. Solving equations is not difficult once you know the proper steps to follow. On the TEAS Mathematics exam, you must be able to solve different kinds of mathematical equations with one variable.

A **variable** is a term that stands for a number or quantity. Any letter can be used for a variable in algebra, but x, y, z, a, b, and c are used most frequently.

A **constant** is a number that is not linked to a variable.

An **expression** is a mathematical phrase that contains constants, variables, and symbols such as +, −, ×, and ÷. An expression can contain parentheses or other symbols as well. Numbers and variables that are separated by + or − signs are called **terms**. Those that are part of multiplication are called **factors**.

Multiplication can be indicated by ×, •, or *, or by parentheses, as in $(2)(3x)$. It can also be indicated like this: xy, which means "x multiplied by y."

An example of a simple algebraic expression is just the variable *x*. An expression may contain two terms, such as $2a + 3b$, or it can be quite complicated, with many letters, numbers, and symbols.

An **equation** is essentially two expressions that are equal. Usually, a variable is included in one or both expressions. **Solving the equation** means finding a value for the variable that makes the equation true.

Since the two sides of an equation are equal, whatever you do to one side of the equation, you must do to the other side. For example, if you add a number to one side, you must add the same number to the other side.

The goal in solving an equation is to put the variable on one side of the equal sign and its value on the other. You do this by using **inverse operations**. Addition and subtraction are inverses of each other, and multiplication and division are inverses of each other.

Here are some examples of how to solve equations by isolating the variable on one side.

- Solve for *x*: $x + 4 = 10$.

    You must get rid of the 4 on the variable side of the equation. Since 4 is added to the variable, you must subtract 4 on *both sides* of the equation. This results in:

    $$x + 4 - 4 = 10 - 4$$

    $$x = 6$$

    To check, substitute $x = 6$ into the original equation.

    $$6 + 4 = 10$$

    $$10 = 10$$

    The answer checks out, so it is correct.

- Solve for *y*: $y - 3 = 7$.

    Likewise, if a value is subtracted from the variable, you should add that number to both sides. For example,

    $$y - 3 + 3 = 7 + 3$$

    $$y = 10$$

- Solve for *a*: $7a = 14$.

You must get rid of the 7 on the variable side of the equation. Since the variable is multiplied by 7, you must divide (inverse of multiply) *both sides* of the equation by 7.

$$\frac{7a}{7} = \frac{14}{7}$$

$$a = 2$$

To check, substitute $a = 2$ into the original equation.

$$7(2) = 14$$

$$14 = 14$$

- Solve for b: $\frac{b}{3} = 6$.

You must get rid of the 3 on the variable side of the equation. Since the variable is divided by 3, you must multiply *both sides* of the equation by 3.

$$3\left(\frac{b}{3}\right) = 3(6)$$

$$b = 18$$

To check, substitute $b = 18$ into the original equation.

$$\frac{18}{3} = 6$$

$$6 = 6$$

An equation may combine all of the above examples. The thing to remember is that whatever you do to one side of the equation must be done to the other side. Here is a more difficult equation with the same variable on both sides:

- Solve for x: $2x + 5 = \frac{x}{3} + 10$.

First, put all of the variable terms on one side by subtracting $\frac{x}{3}$ from both sides.

$$2x + 5 - \frac{x}{3} = \frac{x}{3} + 10 - \frac{x}{3}$$

$$2x + 5 - \frac{x}{3} = 10$$

Next, to put all of the constant (number) terms on the right-hand side, subtract 5 from both sides.

$$2x + 5 - \frac{x}{3} - 5 = 10 - 5$$

$$2x - \frac{x}{3} = 5$$

Multiply all terms on both sides by 3 to get rid of the fraction.

$$3\left(2x - \frac{x}{3}\right) = 3(5)$$

$$6x - x = 15$$

$$5x = 15$$

$$x = 3$$

To check, substitute $x = 3$ into the original equation.

$$2(3) + 5 = \frac{3}{3} + 10$$

$$6 + 5 = 1 + 10$$

$$11 = 11$$

To solve an equation in one variable, you must understand what a variable is and use inverse operations to solve for the variable in an equation.

M.1.4 PROBLEM 1

Solve the equation $5x = 65$ for x.

(A) 13

(C) $\frac{5}{65}$

(B) –13

(D) $\frac{1}{13}$

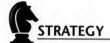

STRATEGY

To solve the equation, apply operations to both sides of the equation in order to isolate the variable on one side of the equation.

THINK

- You want to remove 5, which is the coefficient of the variable.

- To do this, divide both sides of the equation by 5.

$$\frac{5x}{5} = \frac{65}{5}$$

$$x = 13$$

Answer (A) is correct.

M.1.4 PROBLEM 2

Solve the equation $y - 45 = 0$ for y.

(A) $\frac{1}{45}$ (C) 45

(B) -45 (D) 90

STRATEGY

Apply the same operation on both sides of the equation to isolate the variable.

THINK

- To solve, add 45 to both sides of the equation.

$$y - 45 + 45 = 0 + 45$$

$$y = 45$$

- Answer (C) is correct.

M.1.4 PROBLEM 3

Solve the equation $\frac{3}{4}n + 7 = 34$ for n.

(A) $n = 28$ (C) $n = 9$

(B) $n = \frac{1}{36}$ (D) $n = 36$

STRATEGY

Isolate the variable by applying the same operations on both sides of the equation.

THINK

- To solve, isolate the variable using subtraction, multiplication, and division.

- First, subtract 7 from both sides of the equation to isolate the variable.

$$\frac{3}{4}n + 7 - 7 = 34 - 7$$

$$\frac{3}{4}n = 27$$

- Next, put the result in fractional form.

$$\frac{3n}{4} = 27$$

- Multiply both sides by 4.

$$\frac{3n}{4}(4) = 27(4)$$

$$3n = 108$$

- Then divide both sides by 3.

$$\frac{3n}{3} = \frac{108}{3}$$

$$n = 36$$

- Answer (D) is correct.

M.1.5 SOLVE REAL-WORLD PROBLEMS USING OPERATIONS WITH RATIONAL NUMBERS

As a nurse or allied health professional, you often must translate a real-world situation into the correct mathematical equation. Word problems about real-world professional situations include words like *reduction, double, total,* and *distribute* that indicate what mathematical operations are required. On the TEAS exam, you must be able to decide on the necessary operations to solve word problems dealing with rational numbers.

When you approach a **word problem,** read the entire problem very carefully before you try to solve it. Discard irrelevant or unnecessary details as you read. Focus on the relevant information to create an equation for the problem.

Assign a variable to the quantity you are looking for. The variable can be *x, y, n,* or any letter you choose. Write down what that variable represents in the problem.

Look for key words that indicate what operation is needed to solve the problem.

- **Addition:** sum, increase, total, combined, added to, more than

- **Subtraction:** difference, decrease, reduced by, fewer, less than, subtracted from

- **Multiplication:** double, triple, times, of, per, product of, rate, multiplied

- **Division:** half, out of, percent, quarter, distribute, quotient of, divided

Think about how to translate the word problem into an equation. Then solve the equation for the variable and check your answer. Make sure the answer is reasonable. For example, a problem that calls for the amount of time it takes to complete a task should not have a negative number for the answer.

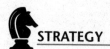 STRATEGY

For a One-Step Problem:

Mrs. Rodriguez's school spends $910 to buy art supplies for the 28 students in her art class. How much does the school spend on art supplies per student?

THINK

The problem is asking what part of $910 each student in art class receives for art supplies. The variable n = each student's share of $910. The equation should read:

$28n = 910$

Solve:

$$\frac{28n}{28} = \frac{910}{28}$$

$$n = 32.50$$

Each student received $32.50 in funding for art supplies.

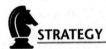 ## STRATEGY

For a Two-Step Problem:

So far this season, Sandra has scored three times the number of goals she scored all last season. If she scores two more goals this season, she will have 20. How many goals did Sandra score last season?

THINK

The problem is asking how many goals Sandra scored last season. So the variable x = number of goals last season. This season Sandra has scored $3x$ goals, or 3 times the number she scored last year. If she scores 2 more goals, she will reach 20 total goals. The equation should read:

$$3x + 2 = 20$$

Solve:

$$3x + 2 - 2 = 20 - 2$$

$$3x = 18$$

$$\frac{3x}{3} = \frac{18}{3}$$

$$x = 6$$

Sandra scored six goals last season.

Check:

$$3(6) + 2 = 20$$

$$18 + 2 = 20$$

$$20 = 20$$

REMEMBER

To solve a real-world problem with rational numbers, you must read the problem carefully, note relevant information, and choose the correct operations and sequence of steps to solve the problem.

M.1.5 PROBLEM 1

Greg had $105 in his savings account. After depositing two identical weekly paychecks, he had $563 in the account. How much money does Greg earn each week?

(A) $105

(C) $359

(B) $229

(D) $458

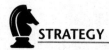

STRATEGY

To solve this problem, find x, the amount of Greg's weekly paycheck.

THINK

- When you subtract the total amount of Greg's two paychecks ($2x$) from $563, you get $105.

- Write an equation for this situation:

  $$563 - 2x = 105$$

- Solve for x:

  $$-563 + 563 - 2x = 105 - 563$$

  $$-2x = -458$$

  $$(-1)-2x = -458(-1)$$

$$2x = 458$$

$$x = 229$$

- Greg's weekly paycheck is \$229. (B) is correct.

M.1.5 PROBLEM 2

Julio's rock garden measures 8 feet by 4 feet. Julio wants to create a continuous border around the rock garden using square concrete paving blocks that measure 6 inches on a side. How many paving blocks should Julio purchase?

(A) 24	(C) 52
(B) 48	(D) 96

 STRATEGY

To solve this problem, first find n, the number of paving blocks needed for the rock garden's perimeter.

THINK

- The total perimeter of the rock garden is $2(8 + 4)$.

- To convert to inches, multiply the perimeter, which is in feet, by 12: $2(8 + 4) \times 12$.

- Since the square paving blocks are 6 inches on a side, the total needed for the perimeter can be expressed as $6n$.

- The equation for this problem is the following:

$$6n = 2(8 + 4) \times 12$$

Simplify:

$$6n = 2(12) \times 12$$

$$6n = 24 \times 12$$

$$6n = 288$$

$$\frac{6n}{6} = \frac{288}{6}$$

$$n = 48$$

- Finally, add 4 paving blocks for the 4 corners of the rock garden's rectangular border. (You can sketch a diagram to see why these are needed.) That will make the border continuous. 48 + 4 = 52. Julio should purchase 52 paving blocks. (C) is correct.

M.1.6 SOLVE REAL-WORLD PROBLEMS INVOLVING PERCENTAGES

Percentage problems crop up frequently in real-world situations. They can involve anything from salary increases to price reductions. On the TEAS Mathematics exam, you will use the concept of percent of a fixed quantity and percentage increase and decrease to solve word problems.

There are three basic types of percentage problems that all fit the same basic framework. That framework has three parts: PERCENT, PART, and TOTAL.

If the variable, or the answer you are seeking, is the PART that is a certain PERCENT of the TOTAL, the equation is:

$$\text{PART} = \text{PERCENT} \times \text{TOTAL} \text{ or } x = \text{PERCENT} \times \text{TOTAL}$$

If the variable is the PERCENT, the equation is:

$$\text{PERCENT} = \frac{\text{PART}}{\text{TOTAL}} \text{ or } x = \frac{\text{PART}}{\text{TOTAL}}$$

If the variable is the TOTAL, the equation is:

$$\text{TOTAL} = \frac{\text{PART}}{\text{PERCENT}} \text{ or } x = \frac{\text{PART}}{\text{PERCENT}}$$

Here are some reminders about working with percentages.

Quick Tips: Percentages

- Find 10% of a number: Move the decimal point 1 place to the left.

- Find 50% of a number: Divide in half.

- Find 1% of a number: Move the decimal point 2 places to the left.

- Find 25% of a number: Divide in half. Then divide in half again.

- Find 20% of a number: Move the decimal point 1 place to the left to find 10%. Then double that figure to make 20%.

- Find 5% of a number: Move the decimal point 1 place to the left to find 10%. Then find half of that figure to make 5%.

- 100% of any number is the number itself.

Now look at a sample word problem.

Shelley's basketball team has made 120 three-point baskets this season. If Shelley has made 45% of these baskets, how many three-point baskets has she made?

THINK

- This problem is asking for the PART of the TOTAL number. The equation to use is: PART = PERCENT × TOTAL.

    $y = .45 \times 120$

    $y = 54$

- Shelley has made 54 three-point baskets.

- When checking your answer, remember that 45% is less than half, so the correct answer is slightly less than half of 120. Thus, 54 is a reasonable answer.

To solve a real-world problem involving percentages, you must use percent of a quantity or percent increase and decrease to calculate the answer.

M.1.6 PROBLEM 1

Last year, 128 babies were born on the fifth floor of the hospital. This year, 160 babies were born on the fifth floor. What was the percentage increase in babies born on the fifth floor?

(A) 20%   (C) 25%

(B) 28%   (D) 16%

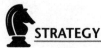
STRATEGY

Create a basic type of percentage framework comparing the increase with the original number.

THINK

- You want to find the PERCENT $= \frac{\text{PART}}{\text{TOTAL}}$.
- The PART is the change, $160 - 128 = 32$. Always calculate change as the new amount minus the original amount. If it is positive, it is an increase; if it is negative, it is a decrease.
- The TOTAL is the original amount, 128.
- So PERCENT $= \frac{32}{128} = .25$, or 25% (answer choice C).

M.1.6 PROBLEM 2

At an electronics store sale, Jasmine purchased a computer tablet that was marked down 23% to $346.50. What was the original price of the tablet?

(A) $450   (C) $875

(B) $506.50   (D) $1,506.52

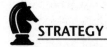
STRATEGY

This problem is asking you to find the TOTAL, or original price before the discount.

THINK

- Use the equation $TOTAL = \frac{PART}{PERCENT}$.

- Now remember that $346.50 is the price after a 23% discount. So $346.50 is 77% of the original price, or total $(100 - 23 = 77)$.

- Plug in the values to write an equation:

$$x = \frac{346.50}{.77}$$

- Solve: $x = 450$

- The original price of the tablet was $450. (A) is correct.

M.1.7 APPLY ESTIMATION STRATEGIES AND ROUNDING RULES TO REAL-WORLD PROBLEMS

As a nurse, you will primarily use metric system measurements in your work. Thus, it is important to be able to estimate these measurements in length, area, volume, and weight. Estimating strategies can also help you solve real-world problems more quickly. On the TEAS exam, you will demonstrate the use of estimation strategies and rounding rules to solve real-world problems.

Remember these approximations for units of measurement in the metric system.

Metric Unit	Real-World Approximation
Gram (g)	weight of one paper clip
Kilogram (kg)	weight of a kitten
Millimeter (mm)	grain of sand
Centimeter (cm)	width of a little finger
Meter (m)	height of a table
Kilometer (km)	12-minute walk for an adult
Liter (l)	contents of a bottle of soda

Estimation is a way of simplifying numbers to make a problem easier to solve. It uses methods of rounding and mental math.

Rounding also is a way of simplifying numbers. For example, a number like 499,732 can be rounded to 500,000 for simpler calculations and to estimate answers.

The method for rounding is to look at the next digit after (to the right of) the place value to be rounded. If it is less than 5, just drop that digit and all the ones to the right (inserting zeros if necessary). If it is 5 or more, add 1 to the digit to be rounded. This method works whether the number is a whole number or a decimal. You only have to know which digit is being rounded.

For example, you can round 1,362 to the nearest hundred. First, look at the 6—the digit to the right of 3, which is in the hundreds place. Since 6 > 5, you change the 3 to 4 and fill in zeros for the rest of the placeholders. So 1,362 rounded to the nearest hundred is 1400.

You can also round fractions and mixed numbers. To round a mixed number to the nearest whole number, check the numerator of its fraction. If the numerator is equal to or greater than half the fraction's denominator, you should round up. If it is less than half the denominator, you should round down.

For example, for the mixed number $3\frac{3}{4}$ the numerator of the fraction, 3, is greater than half of the denominator 4. You should round this mixed number up to 4. For $3\frac{3}{8}$ the numerator 3 is less than half of the denominator 8. You should round this mixed number down to 3.

> *To apply estimation strategies and rounding rules to solving problems, you must know when estimation, or rounding, is appropriate and practice using these strategies correctly.*

Mental math is a term used for any calculation you can do in your head. For example, if you have to distribute 200 pills equally among 10 containers, you know you should not put 30 pills in the first container. You can calculate right away that each container should have 20 pills.

Often mental math is a form of estimation. Suppose you have to distribute 96 pills equally among 6 containers. Your choices are (A) 5 pills per container, (B) 16 pills per container, (C) 21 pills per container, and (D) 43 pills per container. You can eliminate answer choices (A) and (D) as being too small and too large. But what about the answers 16 and 21? Mental math helps you determine that 21 pills is too large a number because 20 × 6 is more than 96.

M.1.7 PROBLEM 1

What is 2,346 rounded to the nearest 100?

(A) 2,400   (C) 3,000

(B) 2,000   (D) 2,300

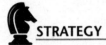

STRATEGY

Circle the **place value** you are rounding to; then look to the right.

THINK

- Because you are rounding to the hundreds place, circle the 3.

- Look to next place value on the right in the tens place. If the tens place digit is 5 or greater, round up. If it is less than 5, round down.

- The 4 in the tens place is less than 5, so round down.

thousands
hundreds
tens
ones

2 ③ 4 6

2 ③ 4 6

2 ③ 0 0

- Write zeros in the places to the right of the number you are rounding.

- 2,346 rounded to the nearest hundred is 2,300. The correct response is (D).

M.1.7 PROBLEM 2

What is 19.796 rounded to the nearest hundredth?

(A) 19.7   (C) 19.79

(B) 19.80   (D) 19.8

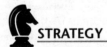

STRATEGY

Circle the place value you are rounding to; then look to the right.

THINK

- Circle the place value you want to round to. Here, you are rounding to the hundredths.

- Look to the next place value on the right.

- The 9 rounds up, so it turns to "10." Write a 0 and carry the 1 to the tenths place, turning the 7 into an 8.

| | | | tens | ones | tenths | hundredths | thousandths |

1 9. 7 ⑨ 6

1 9. 7 ⑨ 6

1 9. 8 ⓪

- 19.796 rounded to the hundredths place is 19.80. The correct response is (B).

- **Key fact:** Always place a digit in the place value you're rounding to, even if it is a zero. The value 19.80 is different from 19.8 because it tells you that the number is accurate to the hundredths place, not just the tenths place.

You can eliminate answer choices (A) and (D) because they are expressed to the nearest tenth, not the nearest hundredth.

M.1.7 PROBLEM 3

A 4,324-lb truck needs to carry a load across a bridge with a legal limit of 6,400 lbs. Which of the following would be the largest load that the truck could legally carry on the bridge?

(A) 2,100 lbs

(C) 2,050 lbs

(B) 2,000 lbs

(D) 2,150 lbs

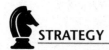

STRATEGY

You don't need an exact answer for this problem. You can use **estimation** to find a sum that is safely less than 6,400 lbs.

THINK

- The weight of the truck plus the load must be less than the bridge's limit. Substituting the known numbers, the weight of the load has to be less than the bridge limit minus the truck weight, or 6,400 − 4,324.

- Do the subtraction to find the maximum weight of the load: 6,400 − 4,324 = 2,076. The answer choice that is closest to this weight without going over it is 2,050, answer choice (C).

- Alternatively, using estimation, by rounding the truck weight to 4,300 pounds, the difference can be figured to be less than 2,100 pounds, so answer choices (A) and (D) are eliminated.

- Of the remaining choices, since the question asks for the largest load, use the larger number, 2,050, and check whether that would be too large: 4,324 + 2,050 = 6,374. Since this is less than the bridge limit of 6,400, the answer is (C): 2,050 lbs.

M.1.8 SOLVE REAL-WORLD PROBLEMS INVOLVING PROPORTIONS

Setting up and solving problems with proportions is an important practical skill for nurses. Proportions enable you to scale dosages up or down as needed, or prepare solutions of a desired strength. On the Mathematics section of the TEAS exam, you must set up and solve real-world problems that involve ratios and proportions.

A **ratio** is a fractional relationship between two quantities.

A **proportion** is a mathematical sentence that states two ratios are equal to each other. When you set up a proportion, be sure that the units for the values in the numerator correspond to each other, and that the same is true for the denominators. In other words, the two ratios should both compare the same two types of things.

Proportions can be written in two ways: $3 : 4 = 12 : 16$ or $\frac{3}{4} = \frac{12}{16}$. These proportions are read as "3 is to 4 as 12 is to 16."

Proportions with variables are called **algebraic proportions**. They are solved by cross-multiplication. This means that you multiply in the form of a cross (×)—each numerator times the opposite denominator. The two products are equal. Thus, for the proportion $\frac{a}{b} = \frac{c}{d}$, cross-multiplication yields the equation $ad = bc$.

Here is a proportion with a variable x. You can solve it by cross-multiplying.

$$\frac{20}{50} = \frac{30}{x}$$

$$20x = 30 \times 50$$

$$20x = 1{,}500$$

$$\frac{20x}{20} = \frac{1{,}500}{20}$$

$$x = 75$$

REMEMBER

To solve a real-world problem involving proportions, you must set two ratios in fraction form equal to each other and solve for the variable.

M.1.8 PROBLEM 1

A nurse adds 4 g of salt to 20 ml of water to make a saline solution. How much salt should be added to 75 ml of water to make a solution of the same strength?

(A) 0.25 g

(B) 10 g

(C) 15 g

(D) 150 g

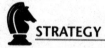

STRATEGY

Use a ratio and a proportion to solve the problem.

THINK

- Here the ratio is 4 g salt to 20 ml water, or 1 to 5.

$$4 : 20 = 1 : 5 = \frac{1}{5}$$

- Write n for the unknown quantity of salt.

$$\frac{1\,\text{g salt}}{5\,\text{ml water}} = \frac{n\,\text{g salt}}{75\,\text{ml water}}$$

- Cross-multiplying as shown
  yields a simple equation,
  $5n = 75$.

$$\frac{1}{5} \not\times \frac{n}{75}$$
$$5n = 75$$
$$n = 15$$

- Solve the equation in the
  normal way. The nurse
  would need 15 g of salt,
  or answer choice (C).

M.1.8 PROBLEM 2

Tamara reads 40 pages of a novel in 52 minutes. How long will it take her to read a novel of 200 pages?

(A) 2 hours, 40 minutes

(C) 4 hours, 10 minutes

(B) 3 hours, 50 minutes

(D) 4 hours, 20 minutes

STRATEGY

Set up a proportion with ratios of pages/minutes to solve the problem.

THINK

- The proportion should be $40 : 52 = 200 : n$. The variable n represents the time it takes Tamara to read 200 pages.

- Cross-multiply to get $40n = 200 \times 52$.

- Then solve: $40n = 10{,}400$.

$$\frac{40n}{40} = \frac{10{,}400}{40}$$

$$n = 260$$

- The answer, 260, represents number of minutes. Convert to hours and minutes: 260 minutes = 4 hours, 20 minutes. Answer (D) is correct.

REMEMBER

An easier way to solve the problem is to look for mathematical relationships. You know that $40 \times 5 = 200$, so the number of minutes Tamara needs to read the novel is 5×52, or 260.

M.1.9 SOLVE REAL-WORLD PROBLEMS INVOLVING RATIOS AND RATES OF CHANGE

Proportions are often used to solve problems involving ratios and rates. How many calories a serving of food has, how many miles a vehicle goes per gallon[†] of fuel, how much money a job pays per hour—these are all rate problems that are fairly easy to solve. On the TEAS, you must solve real-world problems involving ratios and rates of change.

A **rate** is a ratio expressed with numbers and units: $\frac{5 \text{ tablespoons}}{2 \text{ quarts}}$. A **unit rate** is a rate expressed as a quantity of one: $\frac{300 \text{ calories}}{1 \text{ serving}}$, $\frac{26 \text{ miles}}{1 \text{ gallon}}$.

A word problem on rate is solved by using a proportion. For example: A typist can type 80 words in 60 seconds. How many seconds would it take this typist to type 200 words?

$$\text{Set up the proportion:} \quad \frac{80}{60} = \frac{200}{x}$$

$$\text{Solve for } x: \quad 80x = 60 \times 200$$

$$80x = 12,000$$

$$\frac{80x}{80} = \frac{12,000}{80}$$

$$x = 150 \text{ seconds}$$

Rate of change can also be used to compare two points on a graph, or two points that each have an x-coordinate and a y-coordinate. The x-coordinate is a number along the horizontal axis of the graph. The y-coordinate is a number along the vertical axis. Rate of change is measured as the **slope** of the line between two points on the graph. Slope is equal to the change in the y-coordinates divided by the change in the x-coordinates. Slope can thus be expressed as $m = \frac{y_2 - y_1}{x_2 - x_1}$. It can also be expressed as $\frac{\text{rise}}{\text{run}}$, or the change in vertical position over the change in horizontal position.

[†] or, for electric vehicles, miles per gallon of gasoline-equivalent (MPGe).

To solve a real-world problem that involves rate of change, you must compare two ratios to describe how one thing changes in relation to something else.

M.1.9 PROBLEM 1

Renay rode her bike 3.2 miles in 12 minutes. At this rate, how long will it take her to ride the entire 42-mile trip from her house to Santa Fe?

(A) 157.5 min

(B) 1.57 hr

(C) 217 min

(D) 2.57 hr

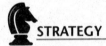

STRATEGY

Use a proportion to solve the problem.

THINK

- Renay's speed can be expressed as a ratio: 3.2 miles to 12 minutes. Express the ratio as a fraction.

$$\frac{3.2}{12}$$

- Set up a proportion using the ratio above and the 42-mile distance to Santa Fe.

$$\frac{3.2 \text{ miles}}{12 \text{ min}} = \frac{42 \text{ miles}}{n \text{ min}}$$

$$\frac{3.2}{12} \diagdown \frac{42}{n}$$

- Solve as you would normally. It would take 157.5 minutes to ride to Santa Fe, making answer choice (A) the correct response.

$$3.2n = (42)(12)$$

$$n = \frac{(42)(12)}{3.2}$$

$$n = 157.5 \text{ minutes}$$

- **Key fact:** In a proportion, make sure that units correspond. Here, for example, both numerators have miles, and both denominators have minutes.

M.1.9 PROBLEM 2

Look at the graph below.

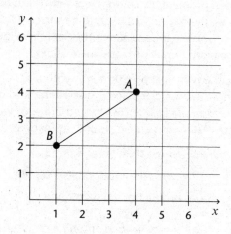

What is the slope of the line *AB*?

(A) $\frac{1}{3}$ (C) 2

(B) $\frac{2}{3}$ (D) 3

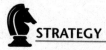

STRATEGY

Use the formula for slope, or rate of change, to solve this problem.

THINK

- The formula for slope is $m = \frac{y_2 - y_1}{x_2 - x_1}$.
- The coordinates for point *A* are (4, 4). The coordinates for point *B* are (1, 2). Plug the *x* and *y* coordinates into the formula.

  $m = \frac{4 - 2}{4 - 1}$

- Simplify: $m = \frac{2}{3}$. The slope of the line AB is $\frac{2}{3}$. Answer (B) is correct.

M.1.10 TRANSLATE PHRASES AND SENTENCES INTO EXPRESSIONS, EQUATIONS, AND INEQUALITIES

A word problem based on a real-world situation must be translated into mathematical language to be solved. On the TEAS Mathematics exam, you must translate written language into mathematical expressions, equations, and inequalities.

A mathematical **expression** is a symbol or combination of symbols to show numbers, variables, operations, and grouping. Examples of expressions include x, $(5 - x)$, and $2(5 - x)$. Words in problems can be translated into an expression, as follows.

nine more than twice a number	$2n + 9$
seven less than four times a number	$4x - 7$
the product of a number and 25	$25y$
thirty-two divided among a number t	$\dfrac{32}{t}$

An **equation** is a statement that two expressions are equal. Word problems can be translated into equations to be solved.

Two fewer than seven times a number equals forty-seven.	$7n - 2 = 47$
Dividing 975 by a number results in 162.5.	$\dfrac{975}{x} = 162.5$

An **inequality** is a statement that two expressions are unequal. Word problems can also be translated into inequalities to be solved.

A number divided by six is greater than 17.	$\dfrac{n}{6} > 17$
Three times a number is less than 124 divided by four.	$3x < \dfrac{124}{4}$

REMEMBER

To translate a word problem into expressions, equations, and inequalities, read the problem carefully and look for key words that tell the quantities, operations, and variables.

M.1.10 PROBLEM 1

Sergio had twelve fewer credits than five times what Joanna had. Which of the following expressions describes the number of Sergio's credits?

(A) $12x - 5$

(C) $5(12x)$

(B) $5x + 12$

(D) $5x - 12$

 STRATEGY

Joanna's number of credits is unknown. It should be written as the variable x.

THINK

- "Twelve fewer" translates to -12.

- "Five times what Joanna had" translates to $5x$.

- The expression for the number of Sergio's credits is $5x - 12$. Answer choice (D) is correct.

M.1.10 PROBLEM 2

Ninety-two dollars added to five times Herbert's weekly salary is less than Mrs. Morton's weekly salary of $1,119. Which of the following describes this situation?

(A) $5s - 92 > 1,119$

(C) $(5s)92 < 1,119$

(B) $5s + 92 < 1,119$

(D) $92 - s > \dfrac{1,119}{5}$

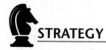 **STRATEGY**

Set up this problem as an inequality between the two weekly salaries.

THINK

- "Five times Herbert's weekly salary" translates to $5s$. Ninety-two dollars added to this is $5s + 92$.

- The expression above is less than Mrs. Morton's weekly salary. The symbol for "less than" is $<$. The inequality should be $5s + 92 < 1{,}119$. Answer choice (B) is correct.

M.2 MEASUREMENT AND DATA

M.2.1 INTERPRET RELEVANT INFORMATION FROM TABLES, CHARTS, AND GRAPHS

In nursing and the allied health professions, you will see a wide variety of graphics: tables, charts, and graphs that convey all kinds of information. To use this data, you must understand how to read different kinds of graphics. On the TEAS, you will demonstrate the ability to read and interpret relevant data from tables, charts, and graphs.

A **line graph** displays a number of data points plotted on an axis grid and connected with lines. Line graphs are often used to show changes over time.

A **bar graph** uses vertical or horizontal bars on a grid to show changes over time or to compare quantities. For example, a bar graph could show the annual number of births in the U.S. from 2012 to 2022.

A **table** presents data arranged in rows and columns. For example, a table might list the number of goals each player on a soccer team scored during the season.

A **circle graph** (or pie chart) presents data as portions of a circle, or percentages of a whole. For example, a circle graph could show how much of a school's athletic budget goes to each sports team.

Always read the title of a table, chart, or graph to see what data it presents. Also read the labels on the horizontal and vertical axes. Look for a **legend**, which explains the data used in the graphic.

To interpret information from tables, charts, and graphs, you must understand how each kind of graphic is set up and what it is designed to do.

M.2.1 PROBLEM 1

The circle graph shows time allocation in hours for nurses on Floor 3 at the Sound Shore Hospital. Use this graph for the following two problems.

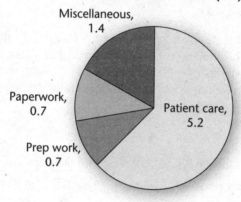

Sound Shore Hospital:
Nurse Time Per Shift (hrs)

What percentage of the time do nurses spend on prep work and paperwork?

(A) 12%

(B) 36%

(C) 17.5%

(D) 48.5%

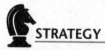

STRATEGY

Use the data in the graph and the proportion method of finding percentages to solve the problem.

THINK

- Add to find the total number of hours in a shift: 8 hr.

Total = 5.2 + 0.7 + 0.7 + 1.4
= 8 hr

- Find the total amount of time spent on paperwork and prep work: 1.4 hr.

Paperwork
+ prep = 0.7 + 0.7
= 1.4 hr

- Use a proportion to find the percentage of time spent doing prep work and paperwork: 1.4 out of 8 = 17.5% (Choice (C)).

$$\frac{1.4 \text{ hr}}{8.0 \text{ hr}} = n$$

M.2.1 PROBLEM 2

A nursing textbook states that nurses in a good-quality facility will spend at least 60% of their time in patient care, but in the best facilities, nurses devote over 70% of their time to patient care. What can you conclude about Sound Shore Hospital from the graph on the previous page?

(A) The hospital rates are substandard.

(B) The hospital is rated good but not the best.

(C) Sound Shore rates among the best hospitals.

(D) Sound Shore rates above even the best hospitals.

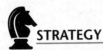 STRATEGY

Find the amount of time in percentage devoted to patient care using the equation method of finding percentages.

THINK

- Find the percentage.

$$\frac{\text{PART}}{\text{TOTAL}} = \text{PERCENT}$$

- Evaluate the percentage. Sound Shore qualifies as good but not the best because it is more than 60% but less than 70%, making (B) the correct answer choice.

$$\frac{5.2}{8.0} = n$$

$$n = 65\%$$

M.2.2 EVALUATE THE INFORMATION IN DATA SETS, TABLES, CHARTS, AND GRAPHS USING STATISTICS

A data distribution shows how data points are clustered or spread out on a graph. This enables you to identify important trends in the data. On the TEAS Mathematics exam, you must analyze trends in data and be able to calculate measures of central tendency.

The **measures of central tendency** (mean, median, and mode) tell you something about the trend of the data.

The **mean** is the average value of the data, and it gives an idea of a typical value. To calculate the mean, add all of the data points and divide by the number of data points.

The **median** is the middle value in a set of data. It is the value at which half the data points are above and half are below. To find the median, put the data in order from smallest to largest and pick the data point that is in the middle. If there are two points in the middle, add them together and divide by 2.

The **mode** is the most frequent value in the data set. Be sure to use the value, not the number of times it appears.

All three measures tell something important about the data set, but they emphasize different things. Which one is used by statisticians (or news reporters) depends on the situation or the point the person is trying to make.

Data can also be displayed on a graph as a **data distribution** of points. The **spread** in a data distribution is the range of values. Typically data is distributed symmetrically in a bell curve, with data points clustered in a single peak in the middle, with fewer points to either side of the peak. Isolated data points that do not fit with the other data are called **outliers**. These are unexpected values that depart from the expected trend of the data.

A **unimodal** data distribution has one clear peak of values. A **bimodal** distribution has two clear peaks.

To use statistics to evaluate data in graphics, you must employ measures of central tendency, which include mean, median, and mode.

M.2.2 PROBLEM 1

The table below shows Hector's scores from seven different judges in a gymnastics competition. Use this table to answer the next two questions.

Judge	1	2	3	4	5	6	7
Score	8.6	7.8	8.6	8.2	9.5	8.6	9.6

M.2.2 PROBLEM 2

Which is greater, Hector's median score or mode score? By how much?

(A) The mode was 0.15 greater than the median.

(B) The mode and median were both the same, 8.6.

(C) The mode was 0.15 less than the median.

(D) The mode was 0.5 greater than the median.

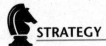

STRATEGY

Identify the mode and median in the data set. Then compare the two values.

THINK

- The **median** is the value that appears as the central value in the data set when it is arranged from least to greatest.

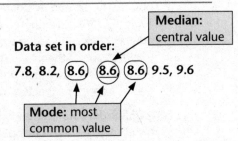

- So 8.6 is the median.

- The **mode** is the value that appears most frequently in the data set.

- So 8.6 is the mode because it appears three times.

- The median and mode are the same for this data set, 8.6, meaning that answer choice (B) is the correct response.

M.2.2 PROBLEM 3

Which score change would push the mean value of Hector's scores to 9.0 or above?

(A) Judge 1 increasing her score to 9.5.

(B) Judge 2 increasing his score by 2.1.

(C) Judge 5 decreasing her score by 0.5 to 9.0.

(D) Judge 2 increasing his score to 9.5.

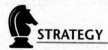 **STRATEGY**

The **mean** is the average score. Find the mean by adding to get the total of all scores and dividing by the number of scores. Find a score change that will result in a new mean of 9.0.

THINK

- Add to find the current total. Divide by 7 to get the mean: 8.7

  Mean: 8.6 + 7.8 + 8.6 + 8.2 + 9.5 + 8.6 + 9.6 = 60.9
  60.9 ÷ 7 = 8.7

- Now find the total that will yield a mean of 9.0

  Mean of 9.0: total ÷ 7 = 9.0
  $n ÷ 7 = 9.0 \longrightarrow n = 63$

- Finally, find the answer choice that will increase the total by (63.0 − 60.9 = 2.1) points.

- Answer choice (B) is the correct response.

- **Check:** Increasing Judge 2's score by 2.1 gives a mean of 9.0.
  Judge 2: 7.8 + 2.1 = 9.9

  Mean: 8.6 + 9.9 + 8.6 + 8.2 + 9.5 + 8.6 + 9.6 = 63
  63 ÷ 7 = 9.0

M.2.3 EXPLAIN THE RELATIONSHIP BETWEEN TWO VARIABLES

Life is full of examples in which changes in one variable cause another variable to change. As you purchase more groceries, your supply of cash goes down. As you drive more miles, the gas in your tank (or the charge in your electric vehicle's battery) decreases. On the TEAS exam, you must identify independent and dependent variables and how they are related.

An **independent variable** stands alone and is not affected by other variables you are measuring.

A **dependent variable** is affected by changes to the independent variable. For example, in a science experiment, several pea plants are exposed to different levels of sunlight. The lighting levels are the independent variable. The growth rate of the plants is the dependent variable. The dependent variable is what is being tested and measured.

The correlation in changes between two variables is called **covariance**. If both variables increase, there is a **positive covariance**, or positive correlation. The variables are directly related. If one variable decreases as the other increases, there is a **negative covariance**, or negative correlation. The variables are inversely related.

In graphing two variables, the independent variable is plotted on the x-axis and the dependent variable is plotted on the y-axis.

To explain the relationship between two variables, you must describe how changes in one variable affect changes in a second variable.

M.2.3 PROBLEM 1

Which of the following pairs of variables has a negative covariance?

(A) x = number of snowfalls in one winter, y = number of snow shovels sold

(B) x = number of hours Reza works in a month, y = amount of Reza's paycheck

(C) x = time spent running on a treadmill, y = number of calories burned

(D) x = number of customers renting a room in a motel, y = number of rooms available

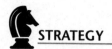

STRATEGY

To solve this problem, remember that negative covariance means that as one variable increases, the other decreases.

THINK

- Answer choices (A), (B), and (C) all show positive covariance. As one variable increases, the other variable also increases.

- For (D), as more customers book rooms in a motel, the number of rooms available decreases. This is a negative covariance, or negative correlation. Answer choice (D) is correct.

M.2.4 CALCULATE GEOMETRIC QUANTITIES

The ability to calculate perimeter and area is a useful everyday skill. You might have to figure how much paint is needed for the dining room ceiling or how many pavers are required to line the front garden. On the Mathematics section of the TEAS exam, you must calculate perimeter and area for various figures, both regular and irregular.

The **perimeter** of a figure is the sum of all the sides. Perimeters are measured in units such as inches or centimeters.

The **area** of a figure is what is enclosed within the perimeter. Area is measured in square units, such as in² or cm². It is a measurement of space within a flat, two-dimensional boundary. **Total surface area** is the sum of the areas of all the surfaces in a three-dimensional object, such as a cube. Total surface area can also measure the surface space of a curved object, such as a sphere or cone.

A **rectangle** is a four-sided figure with four right angles (90°). A rectangle has a length (*l*) and a width (*w*). These opposite sides are equal. Generally the longer sides are designated *l*, but it actually doesn't matter which is called which.

l

w

The perimeter of a rectangle is $l + w + l + w$, or

$$p = 2l + 2w$$

The area of a rectangle is length times width, or

$$A = l \times w$$

A **square** is a special type of rectangle with all equal sides, usually called s, so its perimeter is $p = 2s + 2s$, or

$$p = 4s$$

The area of a square is $s \times s$, or

$$A = s^2.$$

A **triangle** has three sides, a, b, and c, so its perimeter is simply

$$p = a + b + c$$

The area of a triangle is essentially half of the area of a four-sided figure, so its area is $A = \frac{1}{2}lw$. However, it is important that these two measures are perpendicular to each other, not just any two sides. Therefore, the area of a triangle is given as

$$A = \frac{1}{2}bh,$$

where the height of the triangle (h) is any length that extends from a corner to a side (called the base, b) and forms a right angle. Two types of triangles and their parts are labeled below. The small square indicates "perpendicular."

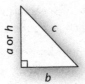
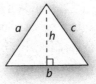

A **circle** is a figure with all its points the same distance from its center.

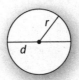

The perimeter of a circle is called the **circumference**. It is calculated as

$$C = \pi d \text{ or } 2\pi r$$

where π is pi (approximately 3.14); d is **diameter**, or the distance across the circle through its center; and r is **radius**, or the distance from the center to any point on the circle. Notice that the circle's diameter is twice as long as the radius. The area of a circle is given as

$$A = \pi r^2$$

Some figures may be made up of several shapes, such as rectangles and triangles. For example, you can calculate the area of a figure such as

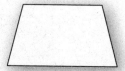

by dividing it into a rectangle and two triangles, if you are given the measurements.

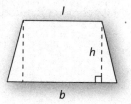

In this case, the two triangle bases are equal and they total $b - l$, so the area is calculated by adding the area of the rectangular part *(lh)* and the areas of both triangles, $\frac{1}{2}(b - l)h$. The total area is

$$A = lh + \frac{1}{2}(b - l)h$$

$$= lh + \frac{1}{2}bh - \frac{1}{2}lh$$

$$= \frac{1}{2}(l + b)h$$

To calculate geometric quantities, you must be able to find the perimeter and area of regular and irregular-shaped figures.

M.2.4 PROBLEM 1

A basketball court has two areas on either end called the keys or free-throw lanes. A diagram of a free-throw lane is shown below.

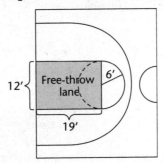

What is the total perimeter measurement of the free-throw lane?

(A) 80.84 ft

(B) 68.84 ft

(C) 56 ft

(D) 87.68 ft

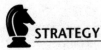 STRATEGY

Add together the perimeter of the rectangular section (minus one side) and half the circumference of the circle.

THINK

- The perimeter of the three sides of the rectangular section is $19 + 19 + 12 = 50$. (The other side that measures 12 is not included.)

- Now you need a perimeter measurement for half the circle. The circle has a radius of 6. So half the circumference is

$$\frac{2\pi r}{2} = \frac{2\pi 6}{2} = \pi 6 = 3.14 \bullet 6 = 18.84$$

- Add 50 + 18.84 = 68.84. The total perimeter of the free-throw lane is 68.84 ft. Answer choice (B) is correct.

M.2.4 PROBLEM 2

What is the total area of the free-throw lane in the diagram on the previous page?

(A) 228 ft²

(C) 284.52 ft²

(B) 248.52 ft²

(D) 341.04 ft²

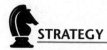

STRATEGY

Add together the areas of the rectangular section and the half circle.

THINK

- Use the formula for area to find the area of the rectangular section of the free-throw lane.

$A = l \times w$

$= 19 \times 12 = 228$

- Then find the area of the half circle, which is $\frac{1}{2}(\pi \bullet r^2)$.

$$= \frac{1}{2}(\pi \bullet 6^2)$$

$$= \frac{1}{2}(\pi \bullet 36)$$

$$= \frac{1}{2}(113.04)$$

$$= 56.52$$

- Add the two areas together: 228 + 56.52 = 284.52. The total area of the free-throw lane is 284.52 ft². Answer choice (C) is correct. Notice that answer choice (D) is incorrect because it includes the area of the whole circle plus the area of the rectangle.

M.2.4 PROBLEM 3

What is the area of the figure below?

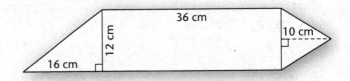

(A) 526 cm²   (C) 696 cm²

(B) 574 cm²   (D) 588 cm²

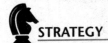

STRATEGY

Use the formulas for areas of a rectangle and triangle to find the total area.

THINK

- First use the formula $A = l \times w$ to find the area of the rectangle: $A = 12 \times 36 = 432$ cm².

- Then use the triangle formula, $A = \frac{1}{2}b \times h$, to find the area of the triangle on the left. Use 16 cm as its base and 12 cm as its height: $A = \frac{1}{2}(16 \times 12) = 96$ cm².

- Use the triangle formula a second time to find the area of the triangle on the right. Use 12 cm as its base and 10 cm as its height: $A = \frac{1}{2}(12 \times 10) = 60$ cm².

- Add the three areas to get the total area: $A = 432$ cm² + 96 cm² + 60 cm² = 588 cm². This makes (D) the correct answer choice.

M.2.4 PROBLEM 4

If this glass aquarium were three-quarters full, how many cubic inches of water would it contain?

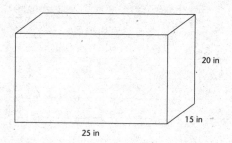

20 in

15 in

25 in

(A) 7,500

(C) 5,625

(B) 6,250

(D) 1,800

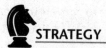

STRATEGY

Use the formula for volume of a rectangular prism to find the total volume. Then multiply that number by 0.75 to find three-quarters of the total volume.

THINK

- First use the formula $V = l \times w \times h$ to find the total volume of the rectangular aquarium. $V = 25 \times 15 \times 20 = 7,500$.

- Then multiply the total volume by three-quarters or 0.75. $7,500 \times 0.75 = 5,625$.

- (C) is the correct answer choice.

M.2.5 CONVERT WITHIN AND BETWEEN STANDARD AND METRIC SYSTEMS

A nurse must deal accurately with units of measurement every day. A mistake in converting between standard and metric units could endanger a patient's health and safety. On the exam, you must demonstrate the ability to convert units within and between the standard and metric systems of measurement.

The system of measurement commonly used in the United States is the **standard system**. (It is also called United States customary units.) The standard system is summarized in the chart below.

Standard System of Measurement		
Length	**Weight**	**Volume**
12 inches = 1 foot	16 ounces = 1 pound	1 cup = 8 fluid oz
3 ft = 1 yard	2,000 lbs = 1 ton	1 pint = 2 cups
5,280 ft = 1 mile		1 quart = 2 pints
		1 gallon = 4 quarts

The standard system has various conversions (seemingly unrelated), and therefore, you must refer to a table such as the one above for conversion.

The measurement system used by most countries in the world is the **metric system**. This system is based on 10s, the same as decimals, so you often need only move the decimal point to convert between measurement units. The metric system is summarized in the chart below.

Metric System of Measurement		
Length	**Weight**	**Volume**
1,000 millimeters = 1 m	1,000 milligrams = 1 g	1,000 milliliters = 1 ℓ
100 centimeters = 1 m	100 centigrams = 1 g	100 centiliters = 1 ℓ
10 decimeters = 1 m	10 decigrams = 1 g	10 deciliters = 1 ℓ
1 meter = 1 m	1 gram = 1 g	1 liter = 1 ℓ
1 dekameter = 10 m	1 dekagram = 10 g	1 dekaliter = 10 ℓ
1 hectometer = 100 m	1 hectogram = 100 g	1 hectoliter = 100 ℓ
1 kilometer = 1,000 m	1 kilogram = 1,000 g	1 kiloliter = 1,000 ℓ

Sometimes it is necessary to convert between the metric and standard systems of measurement. For example, conversion is necessary when a dosage is given per body weight in kilograms, but the patient's weight is given in pounds.

The chart that follows includes some conversions from the metric system to the standard system.

Metric/Standard Conversion		
Length	**Weight**	**Volume**
1 km = 0.62 mile	28.35 g = 1 oz	1 liter = 33.81 fl oz
1 m = 39.37 in	1 kg = 2.205 lb	3.79 liters = 1 gallon

On the TEAS Mathematics exam, you will see conversion problems like the following:

Betsy has a 2.5-gallon jug of saline solution. How many ml does the jug contain?

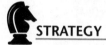

STRATEGY

To solve the problem, you should use a series of ratios and then cancel units.

THINK

- Write the quantity as a fraction: $\dfrac{2.5 \text{ gal}}{1}$.

- Multiply your ratio by another identity ratio (from the table) that cancels with your units. $\dfrac{3.79 \text{ liters}}{1 \text{ gal}}$.

- Multiply by other identity ratios until you obtain the units you are looking for—milliliters.

$$\frac{2.5 \text{ gal}}{1} \times \frac{3.79 \text{ l}}{1 \text{ gal}} \times \frac{1,000 \text{ ml}}{1 \text{ l}} = 9,475 \text{ ml}$$

- 2.5 gallons of saline is equal to 9,475 ml.

To convert between the standard and metric systems, you must know conversion factors and how to calculate equivalent values between measurement systems.

M.2.5 PROBLEM 1

A nurse poured 3.2 quarts of liquid into a container. How many fluid ounces were in the container?

(A) 96 fl oz

(C) 102.4 fl oz

(B) 44.4 fl oz

(D) 202.6 fl oz

STRATEGY

Use a series of ratios to solve the problem. Cancel units.

THINK

- Write the quantity you want to convert as a fraction:
  $$\frac{3.2 \text{ qt}}{1}.$$

- Multiply your ratio by another identity ratio (from the table) that cancels with your units: $\frac{2 \text{ pints}}{1 \text{ qt}}$. Quarts cancel with quarts.

- Keep multiplying by different identity ratios until you reach the units you are looking for—in this case, fluid ounces.

  $$\frac{3.2 \text{ qt}}{1} = \frac{2 \text{ pint}}{1 \text{ qt}} \times \frac{2 \text{ cup}}{1 \text{ pint}} \times \frac{8 \text{ fl oz}}{1 \text{ cup}} = 102.4 \text{ fl oz}$$

- 3.2 quarts is equal to 102.4 fluid oz. So answer choice (C) is correct.

- **Key facts:** Units are the key to conversion problems. Start with the units you have. Keep multiplying by identities to get to the units you want. Note: If the units of your answer are not correct, your answer cannot be correct.

Use common sense and common knowledge to solve problems. For this problem, you may be aware that 1 qt = 32 fluid oz. You can use this conversion identity directly to solve the problem rather than go through a series of conversions.

M.2.5 PROBLEM 2

45.6 cm equals how many hectometers?

(A) 45,600 hm

(C) 0.00456 hm

(B) 0.456 hm

(D) 4.56 hm

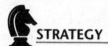

STRATEGY

Move the decimal point using powers of 10 to convert.

THINK

- Start with the units you want to convert: centimeters.

- Count the number of places you need to go to reach hectometers: 4 places.

- Move the decimal point 4 places LEFT to go from centimeters to hectometers.

Length
1,000 millimeters = 1 m
100 centimeters = 1 m
10 decimeters = 1 m
1 meter = 1 m
1 dekameter = 10 m
1 hectometer = 100 m
1 kilometer = 1,000 m

4 places

Decimal point in 45.6 moved 4 places left = 0.00456

$0.0045.6$ cm = 0.00456 hm

- This means that answer choice (C) is correct.

- **Check:** A common-sense check for a conversion problem is of *critical* importance. 45.6 centimeters is about the length from your fingertips to your elbow. So it must be a small fraction of a hectometer, which is 100 m in length.

A centimeter, the size of your fingernail, is much smaller than a hectometer, which is longer than a football field. So you can definitely rule out answer choices (A) and (D) as far too large to be correct.

M.2.5 PROBLEM 3

Each day, a 125-lb patient is supposed to receive 0.8 mg of medication per kilogram of body weight. Which dosage should the patient receive?

(A)   4.56 mg   (C)   45.36 mg

(B)   456.4 mg   (D)   22.5 mg

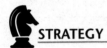

STRATEGY

Write equations to solve the problem, based on the conversion table.

THINK

- Use a proportion to convert the patient's weight to kilograms.

$$\frac{125 \text{ lb}}{n \text{ kg}} = \frac{2.205 \text{ lb}}{1 \text{ kg}}$$

$$n = 56.7 \text{ kg}$$

- Write an equation to find the dose.

$$\text{Dose} = 0.8 \text{ mg/kg} \times \text{wt}$$

- Calculate the dose.

$$= 0.8 \,(56.7)$$

$$= 45.36 \text{ mg}$$

- The patient should receive 45.36 mg of medication, answer choice (C).

SCIENCE

The third section of the TEAS covers Science. It features 44 scored items. There are four categories of Science objectives for the TEAS. The test items are divided among the Science objectives as follows.

S.1 HUMAN ANATOMY AND PHYSIOLOGY—18 SCORED QUESTIONS

S.1.1   Describe the general anatomy and physiology of a human.

S.1.2. Describe the anatomy and physiology of the respiratory system.

S.1.3   Describe the anatomy and physiology of the cardiovascular system.

S.1.4   Describe the anatomy and physiology of the gastrointestinal system.

S.1.5   Describe the anatomy and physiology of the neuromuscular system.

S.1.6   Describe the anatomy and physiology of the reproductive system.

S.1.7   Describe the anatomy and physiology of the integumentary system.

S.1.8   Describe the anatomy and physiology of the endocrine system.

S.1.9   Describe the anatomy and physiology of the genitourinary system.

S.1.10 Describe the anatomy and physiology of the immune system.

S.1.11 Describe the anatomy and physiology of the skeletal system.

S.2 BIOLOGY—9 SCORED QUESTIONS

S.2.1   Describe the basic macromolecules in a biological system.

S.2.2   Describe the structure of cells and the process of cell division.

S.2.3   Describe microorganisms and infectious diseases.

S.2.4   Compare and contrast chromosomes, genes, and DNA.

S.2.5   Explain Mendel's laws of heredity.

S.3 CHEMISTRY—8 SCORED QUESTIONS

S.3.1   Recognize basic atomic structure.

S.3.2   Explain characteristic properties of substances.

S.3.3   Compare and contrast changes in states of matter.

S.3.4   Describe chemical reactions.

S.4 SCIENTIFIC REASONING—9 SCORED QUESTIONS

S.4.1   Identify basic scientific measurements using laboratory tools.

S.4.2   Critique a scientific explanation using logic and evidence.

S.4.3   Explain relationships among events, objects, and processes.

S.4.4   Analyze the design of a scientific investigation.

In addition, the TEAS Science section features six unscored items (aka "pretest" items). These items can address objectives from any of the above categories. You will have 60 minutes to complete the entire Science section.

S.1 HUMAN ANATOMY AND PHYSIOLOGY

S.1.1 DESCRIBE THE GENERAL ANATOMY AND PHYSIOLOGY OF A HUMAN

Anatomy is the structure of the body, while physiology includes the normal functions of a living creature. The human body features a hierarchy (system of levels) of structures and functions that go from the smallest part of a cell to organ systems that nourish or protect the entire body.

On the Science portion of the TEAS exam, you must be able to describe each of these structures and functions. You must also apply correct terminology to describe human anatomical structures and their precise location.

The hierarchy of structures and functions begins with cells. You should know the basic tenets of **cell theory**.

- All living organisms are composed of cells.
- The cell is the basic unit of structure and organization in organisms.
- All cells come from preexisting cells.

Describe how cells carry out **the basic processes of life**.

- Take in food and metabolize it for energy
- Respond to the environment
- Grow
- Reproduce
- Dispose of waste

Remember that, in multicellular organisms such as humans, cells are used as **building blocks** to form more complex body parts.

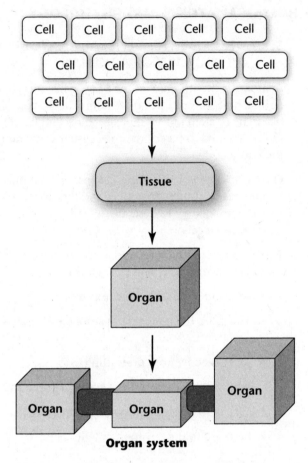

Organ system

Cells that have a specialized function join together to form **tissues**. The four main types of tissue are:

- Connective tissue (bone and cartilage)
- Muscle tissue (skeletal and cardiac muscles)
- Nervous tissue (brain cells and spinal nerves)
- Epithelial tissue (organ surfaces, mouth lining, and skin)

Recognize that tissues join together to form **organs**. Examples of organs include the heart, brain, stomach, and kidneys.

Organs and tissues join together to form **organ systems**. The ten major organ systems in the human body are:

- Respiratory system
- Cardiovascular system
- Gastrointestinal system
- Neuromuscular system
- Reproductive system
- Integumentary system
- Endocrine system
- Genitourinary system
- Immune system
- Skeletal system

These systems work together in a coordinated way to maintain **homeostasis**—a stable environment inside the human body.

To describe the general anatomy and physiology of a human, become familiar with cell theory, the hierarchy of structures and functions, the tissues and their functions, and the organs and organ systems and their functions. Also, know basic anatomical positions and the planes and cavities for the human body.

When preparing for the TEAS, become familiar with the **standard anatomical position** for human anatomy: The body is upright and faces forward; the feet are flat and directed forward; and the upper limbs are held at the body's side with palms facing forward.

Remember the **anatomical planes** for human anatomy.

- **Coronal Plane:** divides body into front and back portions. (Anterior—front, Posterior—back; Ventral—front, Dorsal—back)
- **Sagittal Plane:** divides body into left and right portions.
- **Transverse Plane:** divides body into top and bottom portions. (Superior—head; Inferior—feet)

Remember the **cavities** related to human anatomy.

- **Ventral Cavity:** located on the anterior side of the body; includes the **Thoracic Cavity**, with the lungs, heart, trachea, esophagus, and thymus gland, and the **Abdominopelvic Cavity**, with the stomach, liver, gallbladder, spleen, kidneys, pancreas, and large and small intestines.

- **Dorsal Cavity:** located on the posterior side of the body; includes the **Cranial Cavity**, with the brain, pituitary gland, and twelve cranial nerves, and the **Vertebral Cavity**, with the vertebrae and spinal cord.

S.1.1 PROBLEM

How many different types of tissue does the human body contain?

(A) three

(C) six

(B) four

(D) eight

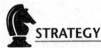 STRATEGY

To answer this question, think about the different types of tissue and their function.

THINK

- Connective tissue, such as bone and cartilage, links the body parts. Muscle tissue, such as skeletal and cardiac muscles, contract to create skeletal movement. Nervous tissue, including nerve cells and fibers, makes up the nervous system. Epithelial tissue comprises the linings of the body's internal and external surfaces.

- These are the four main types of tissue in the human body. Answer (B) is correct.

S.1.2 DESCRIBE THE ANATOMY AND PHYSIOLOGY OF THE RESPIRATORY SYSTEM

On average, a person breathes about 20,000 times a day. Breathing involves taking in oxygen from the surrounding air and releasing carbon dioxide as a waste gas. The respiratory system manages this process, which the body's cells require for energy and growth.

On the TEAS exam, you must be able to describe the parts of the respiratory system and how they work together to keep the cells healthy and provided with energy.

The function of **respiration** is to provide oxygen to the body cells for use in creating energy. This is accomplished through **gas exchange** to the cells, delivering oxygen and removing carbon dioxide as waste. The lungs and the respiratory system perform the gas exchange process automatically.

To describe the anatomy and physiology of the respiratory system, become familiar with the specific parts of the system and how it functions to move oxygen into the body's cells and move carbon dioxide out of the cells.

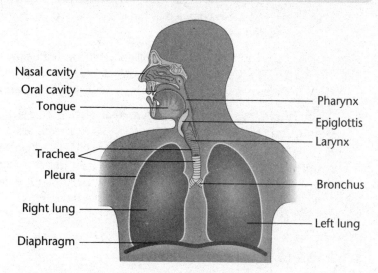

The gas exchange process takes place as follows:

- Air is inhaled from the atmosphere and enters the nose. Air passes through the nasal cavity, **pharynx**, and **larynx**.

- From the larynx, air enters a cartilage-lined tube called the **trachea**. The **epiglottis** is a flap that covers the trachea and prevents solid and liquid material from entering it when you swallow.

- The trachea divides into two **bronchi** that go to the lungs. Inside the lungs the bronchi branch out into narrower tubes called **bronchioles**. At the end of the bronchioles are small sacs called **alveoli**. As you inhale and exhale, the alveoli inflate and deflate like clusters of tiny balloons. This is the main site of gas exchange.

- The thin walls of the alveoli have an enormous surface area to facilitate gas exchange. If pressed flat and spread out, the alveoli would encompass a football field.

- Gas exchange takes place by diffusion between the alveoli and blood. Oxygen diffuses through the **surfactant**, or fluid coating the membranes of the alveoli. The surfactant reduces the pressure required to inflate the alveoli by lowering surface tension. Oxygen passes through the alveoli wall into the surrounding blood capillaries and into red blood cells.

- When you exhale, the process is reversed. Oxygen and carbon dioxide are exchanged in the alveoli. Carbon dioxide is released as a waste gas.

- The **diaphragm** is a domelike muscle located below the lungs. The diaphragm flattens to draw air into the lungs and expands to force air out.

The **respiratory and the cardiovascular systems** interact by way of the heart and lungs. (The cardiovascular system is also called the circulatory system.) The heart delivers deoxygenated blood through the pulmonary arteries to the lungs. There the gas exchange occurs, with the blood taking in oxygen from the alveolar sacs and releasing its store of carbon dioxide. The oxygenated blood returns to the heart and is circulated to the rest of the body.

S.1.2 PROBLEM

What symptoms would you expect in a patient with low blood oxygen?

(A) joint pain

(C) excessive bleeding

(B) weakness and low energy

(D) nausea

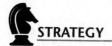

STRATEGY

Refer to the process of respiration to determine how low oxygen would affect a person.

THINK

- Remember that the purpose of respiration is to supply oxygen to cells. This oxygen is used to "burn" food and create energy.

- Therefore, a person with low oxygen would be energy depleted and feel weak. Answer (B) is correct.

S.1.3 DESCRIBE THE ANATOMY AND PHYSIOLOGY OF THE CARDIOVASCULAR SYSTEM

Heart health is a major concern because the heart plays such a vital role in the body's various systems—delivering nutrients, removing waste products, regulating hormones, and fighting infections. On the TEAS exam, you must be able to describe the parts of the cardiovascular system and how they work together to circulate blood and lymph throughout the body.

The function of the **cardiovascular system** (also called the **circulatory system**) is to transport materials to and from the body's cells. Blood is the major carrier of these materials.

The materials the cardiovascular system carries *to* the body cells include:

- **Nutrients** from the digestive system

- **Oxygen** from the respiratory system

- **Hormones,** such as insulin, that are secreted by glands and nerve cells

- **Immune cells** and products that fight infections

The materials that the cardiovascular system carries *away from* the body cells include:

- **Waste products** that eventually get excreted as urine

- **Carbon dioxide** that eventually is exhaled

- **Excess salts and other materials** that are often retained by the body

Arteries are thick-walled vessels that carry oxygenated blood *away from* the heart. Arteries branch into smaller vessels called **arterioles** and then into even smaller vessels called **capillaries**.

Veins are thinner-walled vessels that carry deoxygenated blood from body cells *back to* the heart. The blood first diffuses in the lungs into tiny capillaries and then returns to the heart through **venules** that merge to create larger veins.

The human heart has four chambers—**the left atrium and right atrium** on top and **the left ventricle and right ventricle** on the bottom. (*Right* and *left* indicate the right and left sides of the body.)

> *To describe the anatomy and physiology of the cardiovascular system, become familiar with the specific parts of the system and how it functions to move blood and lymph around the body, distribute nutrients, and eliminate wastes.*

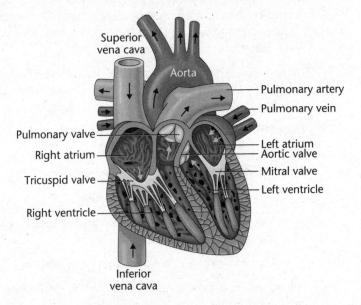

Blood is transported through the body on a system of two loops, or circuits. The **pulmonary loop** transports deoxygenated blood from the right ventricle to the lungs and carries oxygenated blood back to the left atrium. The **systemic loop** transports oxygenated blood from the left ventricle to the body and carries deoxygenated blood back to the right atrium.

The rhythmic contraction and relaxation of heart muscles is called the **heart cycle. Systole** is the contraction of heart muscles. **Diastole** is the relaxation of heart muscles.

The **sinoatrial node**—also called the **pacemaker**—is located in the upper wall of the right atrium and controls heart muscle contractions by sending out electrical signals.

Blood has four main components: plasma, red blood cells, white blood cells, and platelets. **Plasma** is the liquid component of blood and moves blood cells through the body. **Red blood cells,** or erythrocytes, carry oxygen (held in a protein called hemoglobin) from the lungs to the rest of the body and return carbon dioxide to the lungs. **White blood cells,** or leukocytes, are made up of five major types of cells that fight infection in the body. **Platelets** are fragments of cells that facilitate blood clotting.

The **lymphatic system** is a network of capillaries and veins that carry interstitial fluids and waste products through a fluid called **lymph.**

S.1.3 PROBLEM

The systemic loop carries oxygenated blood to the body from which chamber of the heart?

(A) left atrium

(C) left ventricle

(B) right atrium

(D) right ventricle

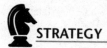

STRATEGY

Refer to the descriptions of the pulmonary and systemic loops in which blood is transported to and from the heart and makes its way throughout the body.

THINK

- In the systemic loop, oxygenated blood travels from the left ventricle to the body. Answer (C) is correct.

S.1.4 DESCRIBE THE ANATOMY AND PHYSIOLOGY OF THE GASTROINTESTINAL SYSTEM

The gastrointestinal system—also called the digestive system—serves to break down food both physically and chemically. Digestion is the process of breaking down food into its molecular components. Essential nutrients in the food are then absorbed into blood vessels and sent on to individual cells.

On the Science section of the exam, you must be able to describe the organs of the gastrointestinal system and how they work together to break down food. You must also know the enzymes and hormones that regulate the digestive process.

The gastrointestinal system begins at the **mouth** and ends with the **anus**. In between, food passes through the **esophagus, stomach, small intestine, large intestine,** and **rectum**.

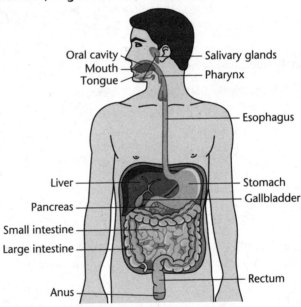

Digestion begins when mechanical chewing and enzymes begin to break down food in the mouth. **Saliva** moistens the food and begins to digest it chemically with enzymes. Food is shaped into a **bolus**, or ball, before it is swallowed.

After being swallowed, food passes into the **pharynx**, or throat. A tissue flap called the **epiglottis** closes the trachea so that food passes into the esophagus.

Food then goes through the esophagus to the stomach. The stomach secretes **gastric juice**, consisting of hydrochloric acid of pH 1 to 2 (highly acidic), the enzyme pepsin, and mucus. Gastric juice serves two main purposes. The acid kills bacteria in the food, and the pepsin digests food proteins. With its folding structure like an accordion, the stomach can store as much as four liters of material. Food mixes with water and gastric juice to make a creamy substance called **chyme**.

Food moves through the digestive system by the muscular squeezing action of **peristalsis**.

The chyme passes through a valve at the stomach's end called the **pyloric sphincter**. This valve regulates passage into the **duodenum**, which is the first part of the **small intestine**. In the small intestine, food is broken down further. Proteins are broken down into amino acids. Starches are broken down into simple sugars.

When broken down to the **molecular level**, food nutrients (sugars, amino acids, and small fats) get absorbed through the walls of the small intestine into the blood. The blood carries these nutrients to the body cells.

Undigested food stays in the small intestine and gets passed on to the **cecum** and into the **large intestine** or **colon**. Water and salt are reabsorbed to create solid waste, called **feces**. This waste is stored in the **rectum**, and is eliminated from the body through the anus.

To describe the anatomy and physiology of the gastrointestinal system, review the specific parts that make up the system and how the system functions to break down food so it can be absorbed and distributed throughout the body.

S.1.4 PROBLEM

Where is food broken down in the digestive system so it can ultimately enter the bloodstream?

(A) in the stomach only

(B) in the stomach, small intestine, and large intestine

(C) in the mouth, stomach, and large intestine

(D) in the mouth, stomach, and small intestine

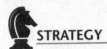

STRATEGY

To answer this question, identify parts of the digestive system that break down food.

THINK

- You should recognize at once that the food that enters the large intestine is not digestible and therefore is no longer broken down for absorption through the small intestine. This eliminates answer (B) and answer (C) because both include the large intestine.

- Enzymes in the mouth begin the process of digestion. Digestion continues in the stomach, and food is broken down to its final molecular level in the small intestine. This means that answer (D) is correct.

S.1.5 DESCRIBE THE ANATOMY AND PHYSIOLOGY OF THE NEUROMUSCULAR SYSTEM

The Central Nervous System

The central nervous system (CNS), which includes the brain and the spinal cord, controls thought and muscle movement in a human being. This enormously complex system transmits signals and impulses that affect every part of the body.

On the Science portion of the TEAS exam, you must describe the parts of the neuromuscular system and how the nervous system exerts control over the muscles.

Neurons, or basic nerve cells, conduct information electrically along incoming **axon** fibers and outgoing **dendrites.** The axon is usually a long extension of the nerve cell body that sends impulses. The dendrite is usually a shorter branched extension that receives stimuli. These stimuli can come from sources such as light (for nerve cells in the eye) or touch (for nerve cells in the hand).

Communication between axon terminals and neurons is done chemically using **neurotransmitters** that are released into the **synapse,** or junction, between neurons.

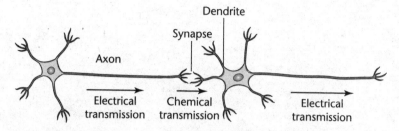

Information is conveyed along the nervous system both electrically and chemically. Axons and dendrites work like electrical wires. Synapses transmit information using chemicals called **neurotransmitters**.

To describe the anatomy and physiology of the neuromuscular system, become familiar with the specific parts of the system and how the nervous system controls voluntary and involuntary muscle movement.

A voluntary movement occurs in the following manner:

- An electrical signal is sent from the brain to a **motor neuron** in the spinal cord.

- The motor neuron relays the signal to the muscle.

- At the muscle, the electrical signal gets transformed into release of the common chemical neurotransmitter **acetylcholine**.

- Acetylcholine stimulates excitable muscle tissue to contract.

The **peripheral nervous system**, a network of sensory nerves that connect to the CNS, is divided into **somatic** (voluntary) and **autonomic** (involuntary) nerves.

Different regions of the brain are specialized for different functions.

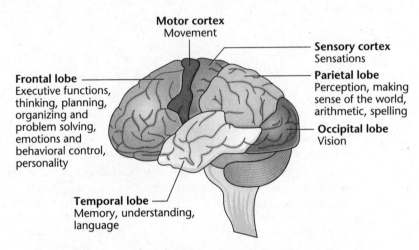

Motor cortex
Movement

Sensory cortex
Sensations

Parietal lobe
Perception, making
sense of the world,
arithmetic, spelling

Frontal lobe
Executive functions,
thinking, planning,
organizing and
problem solving,
emotions and
behavioral control,
personality

Occipital lobe
Vision

Temporal lobe
Memory, understanding,
language

The **cortex**, or outer rind, of the brain, is a layer of tissue about
the thickness of three dimes. The cortex performs the brain's most
sophisticated functions.

Visual information enters the back of the brain in the **occipital lobe**.

Note that the **sensory cortex** is near the **motor cortex** for quick
action.

The planning-reasoning-imagining area of the brain is in the **frontal
lobe**. This is where executive function and decision making largely
occur.

The Muscular System

The **muscular system** enables body movement and maintains
posture. There are three kinds of muscle tissue: **skeletal muscle**,
cardiac muscle, and **smooth muscle**.

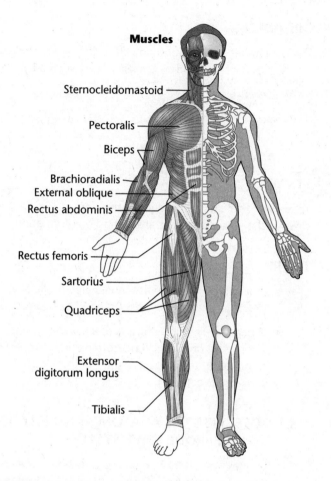

Muscles

Sternocleidomastoid

Pectoralis

Biceps

Brachioradialis
External oblique
Rectus abdominis

Rectus femoris

Sartorius

Quadriceps

Extensor
digitorum longus

Tibialis

Skeletal muscles, which are attached to bones, are the only one of the three types that can be consciously controlled.

Smooth muscles move substances through organs. The digestive system has smooth muscles.

Muscles can only contract; they cannot extend.

Muscles are arranged in antagonistic pairs such as the **biceps** and **triceps**. When the biceps contracts, the triceps relaxes and bends the limb. When the triceps contracts, the biceps relaxes and extends the limb.

Bones are connected to other structures by **tendons** and **ligaments**. Tendons connect bones to muscles, and ligaments connect bones to other bones, usually at joints.

S.1.5 PROBLEM

A patient has been diagnosed with a chemical imbalance in his brain. Which part of his neurons is likely to be affected by this imbalance?

(A) dendrites

(C) synapses

(B) axons

(D) lateral

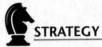

STRATEGY

To answer this question, identify the part of the neuron that is most closely related to chemical transmission of information.

THINK

- In a neuron, the impulse travels electrically along the axon and dendrite, making answers (B) and (A) incorrect choices.

- When the electrical impulse reaches the synapse, it causes the release of chemical neurotransmitters that transmit the information to the next neuron in the sequence. This makes answer (C) correct.

S.1.6 DESCRIBE THE ANATOMY AND PHYSIOLOGY OF THE REPRODUCTIVE SYSTEM

The complex system for human reproduction actually consists of two systems: male and female. Overall, these systems work along with the endocrine system to affect various parts of the body and facilitate reproduction.

On the Science portion of the TEAS, you must identify parts of the male and female reproductive systems and show knowledge of how they function and how they interact with the endocrine system.

The **female reproductive system** includes the following:

- The **ovaries** (singular: **ovary**) are the organs where **ova**, or eggs, are produced.

- The **oviduct**, or **fallopian tube**, is the tube through which eggs move from the ovary to the uterus. Each of the two ovaries has an oviduct.

- The **uterus**, or womb, is where the embryo develops until birth. The fertilized ovum attaches to the **endometrium**, or inside wall, of the uterus.

- The **vagina** is also called the birth canal. During birth, the fetus passes through the **cervix** (the mouth of the uterus) into the vagina, and then emerges from the body.

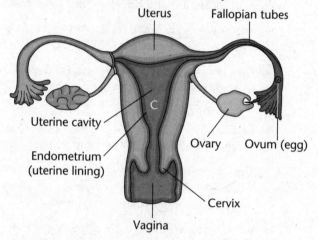

The **male reproductive system** includes the following:

- **Testicles** (or **testes**; singular: **testis**) are the male gonads. Sperm production in the testes takes place in **seminiferous tubules**. The two testes are contained in the **scrotum**, a sac that hangs outside the abdominal cavity.

- **Epididymis** is the coiled tube in each testis where sperm are stored and develop mobility.

- The **vas deferens** is one of two muscular ducts carrying ejaculated sperm from the epididymis to the **urethra**. The urethra, a tube located in the penis, carries semen and urine.

- **Seminal vesicles** are two glands that during ejaculation secrete mucus, fructose, and the hormone **prostaglandin**.

- The **prostate gland** is a large gland that secretes **semen**, a milky alkaline fluid containing sperm and other secretions, into the urethra.

To describe the anatomy and physiology of the reproductive system, become familiar with the specific parts of both the male and female systems and how they function in human reproduction.

Sexual reproduction and development takes place as follows:

- Sperm are made in the testes, whose processes are controlled by the hormone **testosterone**.

- Eggs are produced in the ovaries. Each month a single follicle matures and releases an egg from the ovary. The mature egg, or ovum, enters the fallopian tube.

- **Fertilization** occurs when the sperm penetrates the egg, the sperm and ovum nuclei fuse, and a **zygote** is formed.

- The zygote moves to the uterus, where it implants (in the endometrium) and begins to grow. The growing cells undergo rapid mitosis and become an **embryo**.

- If it fails to be fertilized, the egg will eventually dissolve within the fallopian tube. On the following month, a new egg will descend, and the process will begin again.

The **endocrine system** creates and releases hormones. These chemical messengers regulate most of the systems in the body including the reproductive system. The sex hormones **testosterone, estrogen,** and **progesterone** govern the release of gametes, or reproductive germ cells. In females, they prepare the uterus for supporting the developing fetus and help produce milk for feeding the newborn. Thus, the endocrine system interacts with the reproductive system in many important ways.

S.1.6 PROBLEM

An ovum stays in the fallopian tube for several days without moving. What can you assume?

(A) The ovum is not mature.

(B) The ovum has been fertilized.

(C) The ovum has not been fertilized.

(D) The ovum may be twins.

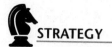

STRATEGY

To answer this question, refer to the steps involved in sexual reproduction.

THINK

- During the first stage of the cycle, the egg matures and moves to the fallopian tube.

- In the fallopian tube, the egg may or may not be fertilized. If it is fertilized, the egg will move on to the uterus. If it is not fertilized, it will stay in the fallopian tube and eventually disintegrate.

- The egg described is not moving, so it must not have been fertilized. Answer (C) is correct.

S.1.7 DESCRIBE THE ANATOMY AND PHYSIOLOGY OF THE INTEGUMENTARY SYSTEM

Human skin, hair, and nails receive enormous attention every day related to grooming and personal care products. But the organs and glands that make up the integumentary system actually play a vital role in protecting the body and regulating body temperature.

On the TEAS exam, you must demonstrate familiarity with the parts of this system and how it works with other systems of the body to maintain healthy function.

The integumentary system is an organ system that consists of **skin, hair, nails, glands,** and **nerves.**

Skin is the human body's outer covering and its largest organ. On average, a person's skin weighs ten pounds and encompasses a surface area of about twenty square feet, yet its thickness is only a few millimeters. Skin makes up a barrier that protects the body from physical damage, ultraviolet light, chemicals, and disease. Skin also helps dispose of bodily waste by sloughing off dead skin cells.

Skin has three main layers.

- The **epidermis** is the outermost layer and is only a tenth of a millimeter thick. About ninety percent of the epidermis consists of cells called **keratinocytes**. The protein keratin makes these cells tough, scaly, and resistant to water. Less than ten percent of epidermal cells are **melanocytes**, producing the pigment

melanin. This pigment protects from ultraviolet rays and
sunburn.

- The **dermis** is the middle layer, consisting of dense connective
  tissue, nervous tissue, and blood vessels.

- The **hypodermis** is the inner layer of loose flexible tissues
  that connect the skin to underlying muscles and bones. The
  hypodermis is also called **subcutaneous tissue**.

*To describe the anatomy and physiology of the
integumentary system, become familiar with the specific
parts of the system and how it functions to protect the body,
regulate body temperature, retain fluids, and dispose of
waste products.*

Hair is an organ of the skin consisting of columns of densely packed
dead keratinocytes. Structurally it has three main parts: the follicle,
root, and shaft. Hair is found in most areas of the body. It serves to
protect the body from ultraviolet radiation and to insulate the body
from cold.

Nails are organs of the skin found on the distal ends of fingers and
toes. Nails are formed of hardened keratinocytes in sheets. They
protect the ends of digits and are useful for scraping or scratching.

Glands in the integumentary system include exocrine glands that
secrete products through ducts.

- **Sudoriferous glands**, or **sweat glands**, secrete water and
  sodium chloride and serve to lower the body's temperature.
  Sweat glands also help remove trace amounts of waste
  products such as ammonia.

- **Sebaceous glands** produce **sebum**, an oily secretion that
  lubricates the skin and makes it more elastic.

- **Ceruminous glands** are found in the skin of the ear canals.
  They secrete a waxy substance called **cerumen** to protect the
  ear canal and lubricate the eardrum.

The integumentary system works with other body systems in various
ways.

- The skin works with the **immune system** by forming a barrier
  or defense mechanism against infection and disease. Oils

secreted by tiny glands in the skin contribute to this function. Immune cells in the skin form a vital first line of defense against infection.

- Surface capillaries on the skin interact with the **circulatory system,** enabling certain substances to enter the bloodstream through capillary networks. Patches that deliver medications (such as nicotine patches for smokers) make use of surface capillaries.

- Capillary networks also work with the **digestive system** by helping to synthesize and absorb vitamin D and promote absorption of calcium in the intestines. Digestion of fats and oils help produce the oils that protect the skin and hair.

- Neurons embedded in the skin work with the **nervous system** to enhance the sense of touch. Inputs from these neurons—such as signals when a hammer strikes your finger—travel to nerve cell connections in the brain that interpret the signals as pain.

S.1.7 PROBLEM

The secretions from sudoriferous glands mainly serve what function?

(A) lubricate the skin for elasticity

(B) cool the body's temperature

(C) protect the ear canal

(D) provide a first line of defense against infection

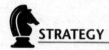 STRATEGY

To answer this question, refer to the functions of the exocrine glands in the integumentary system.

THINK

- Note that sudoriferous glands are also called sweat glands.

- Sweat glands secrete water and sodium chloride to cool the body. Answer (B) is correct.

S.1.8 DESCRIBE THE ANATOMY AND PHYSIOLOGY OF THE ENDOCRINE SYSTEM

The **endocrine system** consists of the body's hormone-producing glands and the hormones they make. (Endocrine glands secrete hormones internally while exocrine glands secrete products outside the body through ducts.)

On the TEAS exam, you must demonstrate knowledge of the endocrine system and how the hormones it produces help regulate certain processes in the body.

The **endocrine system** is made up of a network of glands that produce **hormones**, or chemical messengers, whose functions include the following.

- **Controlling growth**—for example, growth hormone (GH) proceeds from the action of the hypothalamus, an almond-sized portion of the brain located below the thalamus, and the anterior pituitary. The hypothalamus plays a crucial role in bridging the endocrine system and the nervous system.

- **Controlling sexual development**—for example, estrogen made in the ovaries helps the female reproductive system develop; it also controls the menstrual cycle.

- **Controlling metabolism**—thyroxin from the thyroid gland regulates basic metabolic rate, or how fast your body's "motor" runs.

Hormone	Gland	Function
Growth hormone	Hypothalamus and pituitary	Growth
Oxytocin and vasopressin	Hypothalamus	Uterine contractions
Thyroxin	Thyroid gland	Metabolism
Insulin and glucagon	Pancreas	Blood sugar
Cortisol	Adrenal cortex	Stress and metabolism
Estrogen and testosterone	Ovaries and testes	Sex

To describe the anatomy and physiology of the endocrine system, become familiar with the specific parts of the system and how it functions to release hormones that regulate various body processes.

Hormones typically are secreted from a gland and travel through the bloodstream. When a hormone reaches its target, it changes activity, structure, or behavior.

Hormones in the endocrine system regulate the body's healthy function. **Hormone imbalance** occurs when glands produce an incorrect amount of hormones. This results in endocrine-related diseases, which are quite common.

A good example is the hormone **insulin**, which is made by the pancreas and regulates the body's use of glucose (sugar) from carbohydrates.

- When food is eaten and glucose enters the blood, the pancreas releases insulin into the blood.

- Insulin allows cells to take in glucose. Without insulin, the body's cells cannot take in glucose.

- Normally, blood sugar levels rise after eating and then drop as insulin is released and glucose is taken into cells and metabolized.

- A person with diabetes is unable to make insulin. Without insulin, the cells of a person with diabetes are starved for glucose. As a result, the person feels weak even though blood sugar levels remain high.

- People with diabetes must carefully control when and how much insulin to take so they can maintain healthy blood sugar levels.

S.1.8 PROBLEM

Which of the following serves as a vital connection between the endocrine system and the nervous system?

(A) the thyroid

(C) the pancreas

(B) the pineal gland

(D) the hypothalamus

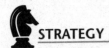

STRATEGY

To answer this question, refer to the functions of the endocrine system and its various parts.

THINK

- The hypothalamus serves as a bridge between the endocrine system of hormone-producing glands and the nervous system. Answer (D) is correct.

S.1.9 DESCRIBE THE ANATOMY AND PHYSIOLOGY OF THE GENITOURINARY SYSTEM

The **genitourinary system**—also called the **urogenital system**—consists of organs involved in excretion, or the process of eliminating bodily wastes. Some of the same structures form part of the reproductive system.

On the TEAS exam, you must identify the parts of the genitourinary system and be able to explain how they work together in the excretion process and the maintenance of homeostasis.

The **genitourinary system** includes the following major structures: **kidneys, ureters, bladder,** and **urethra**.

The key organs for excretion are the **kidneys**. Each kidney is divided into two major parts called the **cortex** and the **medulla**.

- Normal metabolism in cells produces waste products that enter the blood along with carbon dioxide. Before it returns to the lungs for oxygen and the small intestine for food, this blood must be filtered and cleaned.

- Toxins are taken out of the blood in the liver. Blood then goes through the renal arteries to the kidneys. (*Renal* means "related to the kidneys.") Filtering of waste occurs in the kidneys.

- Each kidney has about one million tiny filtering tubes, or **nephrons**. Each nephron tube features a **glomerulus**, a cluster of capillaries that acts like a filter.

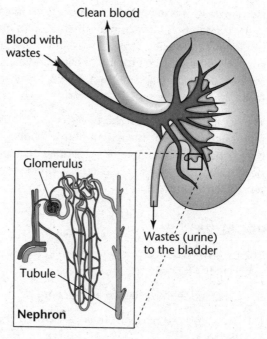

Clean blood

Blood with wastes

Glomerulus

Tubule

Nephron

Wastes (urine) to the bladder

- The nephron actually performs three processes: filtration, secretion, and reabsorption.

- The glomerulus keeps proteins, key ions such as sodium and potassium, and other valuable substances in the body. It allows waste and excess fluid to collect in a tubule. Waste fluid, called **urine**, passes through **ureters** to the **bladder**, where it is stored temporarily. From the bladder, urine exits through the **urethra** and out of the body.

REMEMBER

To describe the anatomy and physiology of the genitourinary system, become familiar with the specific parts of the system and how these parts function together to rid the body of wastes and maintain its balance of salt and water.

Homeostasis is a self-regulating process for maintaining equilibrium in the human body. The genitourinary system maintains homeostasis by eliminating wastes, regulating acidity in the blood, and controlling blood levels for metabolites and electrolytes, including sodium, potassium, and calcium. Kidneys play a vital role in maintaining homeostasis.

The genitourinary system shares ducts and tubules with the reproductive system. The extent of this sharing is greater for males than females. For example, the urethra, which passes through the penis, conducts urine in the excretory process and semen in the reproductive process.

S.1.9 PROBLEM

The cause of advanced kidney disease in a person is most likely which of the following?

(A) The bladder has a bacterial infection.

(B) The nephrons have lost their capacity to filter wastes out of the blood.

(C) The kidneys have lost their elasticity.

(D) Renal arteries no longer supply sufficient blood supply to the kidneys.

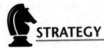

STRATEGY

To answer this question, refer to the structures of the genitourinary system.

THINK

- A bacterial infection is not related to advanced kidney disease. Answer (A) is incorrect.

- Kidneys' loss of elasticity is caused by aging or hypertension, so answer (C) is incorrect.

- Renal artery stenosis is more often the result of chronic kidney disease rather than the cause of it, so answer (D) is incorrect.

- Kidney disease is usually caused by damaged nephrons that do not filter the blood. Answer (B) is correct.

S.1.10 DESCRIBE THE ANATOMY AND PHYSIOLOGY OF THE IMMUNE SYSTEM

Like an army that rallies and closes ranks when faced with an invading force, the immune system provides three lines of defense against disease-causing microorganisms. On the TEAS exam, you must demonstrate knowledge about the parts of the immune system and how the system interacts with the body's other systems.

The **human immune system** is a network of cells, tissues, and organs that work in concert to protect the body from attack by tiny organisms that cause infections.

The immune system consists of three major lines of defense against infections and **antigens** and **pathogens** (agents that cause disease).

The **first line of defense** is nonspecific and forms a barrier that keeps pathogens from entering the body. The skin and assorted body fluids—tears, mucus, saliva, waxes, and stomach acid—keep infections out and can expel them if they enter.

The **second line of defense** is also nonspecific and comes into play when microbes invade the body. This second line attempts to limit the spread of invading microbes before any specific immune response begins. The swelling and redness of inflammation signal that the body has called in white blood cells and natural killer (NK) cells to consume bacteria and destroy body cells infected with a virus.

To describe the anatomy and physiology of the immune system, become familiar with the specific parts of the system and how it functions to protect the body from disease and infection.

White blood cells, or **phagocytes**, "swallow" bacteria that have been identified by helper T cells. **Interferons** combat virus invaders and block cell-to-cell infections.

The **third line of defense** is specific. In other words, its defenses are "custom made" to fight off specific infections. The third line relies on two types of cells that originate in the bone marrow: **B lymphocytes** and **T lymphocytes**.

Antigens (foreign proteins) bind to B lymphocytes or B cells, which produce antibodies specific to that infection. Antibodies are produced at the rate of 2,000 per second. This is called the **humoral response** or **antibody-mediated response**.

The immune system keeps a certain number of lymphocytes, called memory cells, around to "remember" a specific infection. If the infection appears again—even years later—antibody production is quickly ramped up to fight off the invader.

With a vaccine, a weakened form of an antigen is introduced into the body to activate B cells to produce antibodies. If the non-weakened antigen then arrives, the premade antibodies attack it.

T lymphocytes originate in the bone marrow but mature in the thymus gland. They attack pathogens by the **cell-mediated response**. **Killer T cells,** or **cytotoxic T cells**, rove the body seeking out "nonself" cells and mounting a campaign to kill them off. **Helper T cells** help both B cells and killer T cells recognize invaders.

The lymphatic system is largely responsible for bringing antibodies and white blood cells to different parts of the body.

S.1.10 PROBLEM

The humoral response fights infection by doing which of the following?

(A) producing antibodies

(B) ingesting microbes

(C) forming a barrier consisting of various body fluids

(D) creating "memory cells" that remember a specific infection

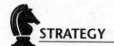

STRATEGY

To answer this question, refer to the three lines of defense of the immune system.

THINK

- You should remember that the humoral response is part of the third line of defense in the immune system.

- Phagocytes swallow, or ingest, bacteria in the second line of defense, so answer (B) is incorrect.

- A barrier of body fluids to prevent infection is part of the first line of defense, so answer (C) is incorrect.

- Creating "memory cells" that remember a specific infection is part of the cell-mediated response, so answer (D) is incorrect.

- In the humoral response, lymphocytes that originate in the bone marrow are activated by specific antigens to produce antibodies that fight the infection. Answer (A) is correct.

S.1.11 DESCRIBE THE ANATOMY AND PHYSIOLOGY OF THE SKELETAL SYSTEM

The skeletal system is made up of bones that support and protect the body's soft tissues and, along with tendons and ligaments, facilitate movement. It can be thought of as the body's scaffold. On the Science section of the TEAS exam, you must demonstrate knowledge of what the skeletal system is and the vital functions it performs.

The **skeletal system** of an adult human is made up of 206 bones and a connective network of tendons, ligaments, and cartilage. Tendons connect bones to muscles, and ligaments connect bones to other bones, usually at joints.

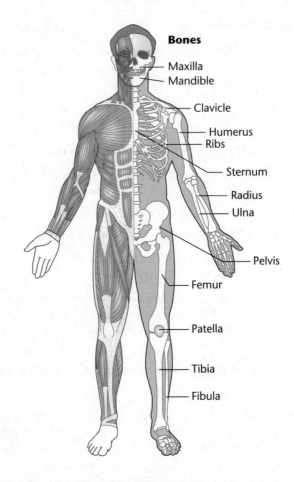

Bones

Maxilla
Mandible

Clavicle

Humerus
Ribs

Sternum

Radius
Ulna

Pelvis

Femur

Patella

Tibia

Fibula

There are four main types of bones: long, short, flat, irregular. Bone is light but very strong. Calcium compounds (such as hydroxyapatite) provide bones with their strength. The protein collagen makes bone flexible.

Bones serve to synthesize blood and immune cells, thus forming a vital connection to the human immune system.

Bones consist of two types of tissue. **Compact bone** is the dense, hard tissue that forms the outer layer of most bones and the main shaft of long bones. Inside the hard tissue of compact bone are nerves and blood vessels. **Spongy bone** (also called **cancellous bone**) is a network of irregularly-shaped sheets making up the inner part of bones. Spongy bone is located at the ends of long bones. It is found in the center of other bones, such as pelvic bones, skull, ribs, and vertebrae. Spongy bone is filled with red bone marrow.

Red bone marrow consists of blood stem cells and blood cells in various stages of development. It creates most of the body's blood cells, including red blood cells, white blood cells, and platelets. It also helps to eliminate old blood cells.

Yellow bone marrow is found in the center of long bones. It mostly consists of fat.

To describe the anatomy and physiology of the skeletal system, become familiar with the major bones of the system and how the system functions and interacts with the neuromuscular system.

Even healthy bones are subject to fracture in accidents or injuries. Diseases of the bones include the following.

- **Osteoporosis** is a disease that causes the bones to become fragile and susceptible to fracture.

- **Leukemia** is a fast-growing cancer of the blood and bone marrow.

- **Arthritis** is a rheumatic disease that can cause pain and stiffness in the joints and progressive loss of bone.

- **Scoliosis** is a bone abnormality that leads to curvature of the spine.

S.1.11 PROBLEM

Which of the following helps to make bones very hard?

(A) red blood cells

(B) collagen

(C) calcium

(D) white blood cells

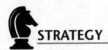

STRATEGY

To answer this question, refer to details about bones and the skeletal system.

THINK

- A calcium compound called hydroxyapatite is responsible for the strength and hardness of bones. Answer (C) is correct.

S.2 BIOLOGY

S.2.1 DESCRIBE THE BASIC MACROMOLECULES IN A BIOLOGICAL SYSTEM

Macromolecules are essential for the human body to carry out life processes. These molecules are based on carbon and contain hundreds or even thousands of atoms. On the Science portion of the TEAS exam, you must show understanding of the structure and function of macromolecules and how these molecules correlate with familiar food groups.

Macromolecules (*macro-* means "large") are large **organic molecules**, or molecules that contain carbon atoms. Four of the six electrons in a carbon atom are available to bond with other atoms, allowing for the long chains or rings of atoms in macromolecules.

Most macromolecules are **polymers**. This means that they consist of a **monomer** (single unit or building block) repeated many times, like a series of beads strung together in a necklace. Monomers join together by covalent bonds resulting from the removal of a water molecule. This is called **dehydration reaction** or **condensation**. The bonds are broken by adding water, a process called **hydrolysis**.

Organic molecules have properties in common because they share similar clusters of atoms. These clusters are called **functional groups**. Each functional group lends a molecule a particular property, such as acidity or alkalinity.

Four types of macromolecules make up all living matter. They are **carbohydrates**, **lipids**, **proteins**, and **nucleic acids**.

Macromolecules			
Molecule	**What It Does**	**Composed of**	**Examples**
Carbohydrates	Energy source	Carbon, hydrogen, and oxygen	Sugars and starches
Lipids	Fats; form cell membranes; used as an energy source	Carbon, hydrogen, and oxygen	Glycerol and triglycerides
Proteins	As enzymes, proteins facilitate chemical reactions that are critical for life processes; structural proteins form muscles, connective tissue	Amino acid chains made of carbon, hydrogen, oxygen, and nitrogen	Pepsin (digestive enzyme), hemoglobin (in red blood cells), and myosin (in muscle cells)
Nucleic acids	DNA makes up chromosomes that code for all proteins	Carbon, hydrogen, oxygen, nitrogen, and phosphorus	DNA and RNA

REMEMBER

To describe the basic macromolecules in a biological system, review the chemical structure and function of organic molecules, including carbohydrates, lipids, proteins, and nucleic acids.

Macromolecules are taken in as food and are essential to nutrition. They correlate to basic food groups as follows:

- **Carbohydrates:** sugars, starches, grains
- **Lipids:** fats, oils, butter, lard
- **Proteins:** meat, beans, leafy green vegetables
- **Nucleic acids:** fish, nuts, fruit

Carbohydrates such as sugars and starches are broken down and "burned" for energy. They are grouped into three categories keyed to the number of **saccharide** (sugar) molecules.

- A **monosaccharide** (chemical formula $C_6H_{12}O_6$) is the simplest carbohydrate, consisting of a single molecule of sugar. Examples are **glucose, fructose,** and **galactose.**

- A **disaccharide** (chemical formula $C_{12}H_{22}O_{11}$) consists of two sugar molecules joined together with a glycosidic linkage. The process of linkage causes one water molecule to be lost (resulting in O_{11} not O_{12}). Examples are **sucrose** and **lactose.**

- A **polysaccharide** consists of monosaccharides connected in a series. Thus, a polysaccharide is a polymer of carbohydrates. Examples are **starch, cellulose,** and **glycogen.**

Lipids are hydrophobic, meaning they are not attracted to water and not soluble in water. They are grouped into three main categories.

- **Triglycerides** consist of fatty acids linked to a glycerol molecule. Examples include fats (saturated and unsaturated) and oils.

- **Phospholipids** are the main ingredient in cell membranes.

- **Steroids** include cholesterol and hormones such as testosterone and estrogen.

Proteins are macromolecules that carry out many important functions in the body. Proteins in food are broken down into amino acids and re-formed into new proteins for muscle and other functions. Proteins are also involved in genetic expression (DNA proteins), structure (keratin in hair, collagen in connective tissue), transport (hemoglobin), digestion (pepsin), immune defense (antibodies), and catalyzing chemical reactions (various enzymes).

Nucleic acids, which include DNA and RNA, are formed from monomers called nucleotides.

S.2.1 PROBLEM

Changing disaccharides to monosaccharides involves which of the following processes?

(A) dehydration

(C) hydration

(B) hydrolysis

(D) condensation

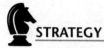 STRATEGY

Think about macromolecules and the relationship of polymers and monomers.

THINK

- To change disaccharides to monosaccharides, you must break the chemical bond by adding water.

- This process is called hydrolysis. Answer (B) is correct.

S.2.2 DESCRIBE THE STRUCTURE OF CELLS AND THE PROCESS OF CELL DIVISION

Distinguish between the two main types of cells: **prokaryotes and eukaryotes**. (For the purposes of this book, archaea and bacteria are grouped together as prokaryotes.)

Prokaryotes	Eukaryotes
Single-celled	Single-celled and multicelled
Bacteria, algae	Plants, animals, fungi, and protists
Extremely small cells	Large cells (10 times as large as prokaryotes)
No nucleus or organelles	Nucleus and organelles
Single, usually circular chromosome	Multiple chromosomes
Reproduces by fission (budding)	Mitosis and meiosis for reproduction and growth

Identify **organelles,** which are the parts of a cell. These membrane-bound structures carry out a cell's basic functions, such as processing food and disposing of waste. Look at the organelles labeled in the cell diagram below. (Eukaryotic cells have organelles, but prokaryotic cells do not.) The diagram is followed by a chart describing the function of organelles.

A Generalized Animal Cell Structure

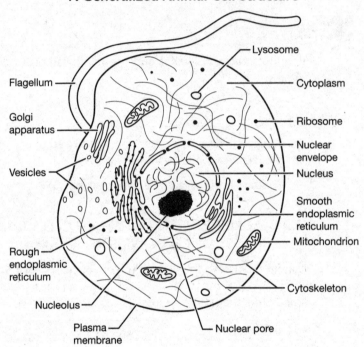

Flagellum

Golgi apparatus

Vesicles

Rough endoplasmic reticulum

Nucleolus

Plasma membrane

Lysosome

Cytoplasm

Ribosome

Nuclear envelope

Nucleus

Smooth endoplasmic reticulum

Mitochondrion

Cytoskeleton

Nuclear pore

Organelles and Their Functions

Structure	What It Does	What Has It
Chloroplast	Site of photosynthesis	Eukaryotic plant cells
Nucleus	Regulates all cell activity, including cell replication; does this through DNA, which codes for enzymes that carry out all important cell "jobs"	All eukaryotes
Ribosomes	Use RNA to transcribe the original DNA code into proteins	Eukaryotes and prokaryotes
Mitochondria	Cell powerhouses; use oxygen to burn glucose and produce ATP for cell's energy	All eukaryotes
Cytoplasm	Watery medium inside of cell	All eukaryotes and prokaryotes
Cytoskeleton	Provides structure for cell and allows for transport	All eukaryotes
Endoplasmic reticulum (ER)	Rough ER has ribosomes and produces proteins; smooth ER used in synthesis of fats	All eukaryotes
Cell membrane	Phospholipid bilayer that acts as a highly selective barrier for passive and active transport.	All eukaryotes and prokaryotes
Cell wall	Stiff outer cell structure	Plants, fungi, and prokaryotes
Golgi bodies	Package proteins; secrete materials outside of cell	All eukaryotes
Vacuoles	Storage containers	All eukaryotes
Flagellum	Locomotion	Prokaryotes and some eukaryotes

Stages of Mitosis	Stages of Meiosis I and II
Interphase: DNA in the cell is copied, resulting in two identical sets of chromosomes	**Interphase:** DNA in the cell is copied, resulting in two identical sets of chromosomes
Prophase: Chromosomes condense into X-shaped structures; mitotic spindle extends across the cell	**Prophase I:** Chromosomes condense into X-shaped structures; mitotic spindle extends across the cell; chromosomes pair up so that both copies of chromosome 1 are together and both copies of chromosome 2 are together; mitotic spindle extends across the cell
Metaphase: The mitotic spindle aligns the chromosomes along the cell's center, or metaphase plate	**Metaphase I:** The meiotic spindle aligns the chromosomes along the cell's center, or metaphase plate; the spindle fibers attach to one chromosome of each pair
Anaphase: Sister chromatids are pulled apart toward opposite poles	**Anaphase I:** Pair of chromosomes are pulled apart toward opposite poles
Telophase: Chromosomes uncoil and a nuclear membrane forms around each set of chromosomes; mitotic spindle breaks down and cytokinesis begins	**Telophase I:** At each pole a full set of chromosomes gather; a membrane forms around each set of chromosomes; meiotic spindle breaks down and cytokinesis begins
	Prophase II: The two daughter cells condense again into X-shaped structures; the meiotic spindle forms again
	Metaphase II: The meiotic spindle aligns the chromosomes (pair of chromatids) along the cell's metaphase plate; the spindle fibers attach to each of the sister chromatids
	Anaphase II: Sister chromatids are pulled apart toward opposite poles; separated chromatids are individual chromosomes
	Telophase II: Chromosomes complete their move to opposite poles of the cell; membrane forms around each set of chromosomes; another round of cytokinesis begins

There are two types of cell division, **mitosis** and **meiosis**. Mitosis, the major type of cell division, is the process of making new body cells. Meiosis is the process of creating sperm and egg cells.

During mitosis, a cell undergoes several stages that result in the duplication of its contents, including its chromosomes. The final stage is **cytokinesis**, in which the original cell splits to form two identical daughter cells.

In meiosis, cytokinesis actually occurs twice. It occurs the first time after the Telophase I stage, producing two identical daughter cells. It occurs the second time after the Telophase II stage. This produces four cells that contain half the original number of chromosomes. These cells—sperm in males, eggs in females—are **gametes**, or human sex cells.

To describe cell structure, become familiar with the organelles and their functions. Study the process of cell division. This includes the stages of mitosis, which produces body cells, and meiosis, which produces human sex cells.

S.2.2 PROBLEM

A patient has a cellular problem that involves protein synthesis. Which organelle is NOT likely to be faulty?

(A) mitochondria

(C) ribosomes

(B) endoplasmic reticulum

(D) nucleus

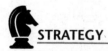 STRATEGY

To answer this question, think about where proteins are made in the cell.

THINK

- Protein production is orchestrated in the nucleus (D) and carried out in the ribosomes (C), Golgi bodies, and endoplasmic reticulum (B). All these organelles could be involved in a cellular problem involving protein synthesis. Thus, all these answer choices are incorrect.

- The mitochondria are involved in metabolism, not protein synthesis, so answer (A) is correct.

S.2.3 DESCRIBE MICROORGANISMS AND INFECTIOUS DISEASES

Infectious diseases are caused by microbes, or **germs**. Germs are found in the air, water, and soil. They are also found inside your body and on your skin. Many germs are harmless and some are even useful. Some, however, can cause illness.

There are four main types of germs:

- **Bacteria** are one-celled germs that are able to multiply quickly. Strep throat, E. coli food poisoning, and tuberculosis are examples of bacterial infection.

- **Viruses** are tiny nonliving infectious microbes consisting of a segment of either DNA or RNA in a protein sheathe. They invade cells in order to multiply. Viral infections include the common cold, measles, hepatitis, influenza, COVID-19, and HIV/AIDS.

- **Fungi** are plantlike organisms, such as mold, mildew, and yeasts. Examples of fungal infections include ringworm and athlete's foot.

- **Protozoa** are one-celled organisms like bacteria. However, they are larger and contain a nucleus and other cell structures, much like plant and animal cells. Some protozoa are **parasites**, meaning they must live on or in another organism.

The **Cycle of Infection** has five components:

- The cycle begins when a **pathogen**, or microorganism, attaches itself to a reservoir host, or living host, such as a person, animal, or insect.

- The second step is the **portal of exit**, or the method by which the pathogen leaves the reservoir host in order to infect another organism. This can include blood, saliva, mucus, or anything from the gastrointestinal or urinary tracts.

- The third step is the **mode of transmission**. This includes droplets (from a sneeze or cough) that reach the recipient's nose or mouth; direct contact with infected blood or saliva, as in sexual contact, or with pathogens on surfaces, such as a doorknob touched by a sick person; and inhalation of airborne particles delivered by air currents. The mode of transmission can also be vector-borne, from vectors such as flies, ticks, mosquitoes, and fleas.

- The fourth step is the pathogen's **route of entrance**, such as a mucus membrane in the nose, mouth, rectum, or vagina.

- The fifth step is a **susceptible host**. This can be someone at higher risk of infection, such as a person with a compromised immune system.

To describe infectious diseases, become familiar with the four main types of germs: bacteria, viruses, fungi, and protozoa. Know the five components of the Cycle of Infection. Also, know the difference between infectious and non-infectious diseases.

Non-infectious diseases are not caused by a pathogen. They cannot be spread from one person to another. Non-infectious diseases include hypertension, asthma, diabetes, cancer, and emphysema.

S.2.3 PROBLEM

Which of the following is characteristic of a virus?

(A) It is alive.

(B) It has a protein coat.

(C) It is composed of cells.

(D) It does not include genetic material.

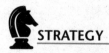

STRATEGY

To answer this question, think about the characteristics of a virus. They are not made up of cells, cannot maintain homeostasis, do not grow, and cannot make their own energy.

THINK

- A virus is nonliving, so (A) is incorrect. It invades cells but is not made of cells itself, so (C) is incorrect. A virus is made of RNA or DNA, so (D) is incorrect.

- A virus features a protein coat or sheathe. Answer (B) is correct.

S.2.4 COMPARE AND CONTRAST CHROMOSOMES, GENES, AND DNA

In 2003, scientists from around the world completed an effort to map all the genes of the human genome—the complete set of genetic instructions. Their work has enabled everything from genetic testing for cancer risks to designs for gene-based medicines. On the TEAS exam, you must demonstrate knowledge of what genes, chromosomes, and DNA are, and how proteins are produced from DNA.

DNA is a nucleic acid. The letters DNA stand for **d**eoxyribo**n**ucleic **a**cid. DNA is the hereditary material in all living things. DNA is located on **chromosomes** in the cell nucleus. Chromosomes are primarily composed of DNA. Each **gene** is a section on a chromosome that codes for a **protein**.

DNA forms a **double helix**, or two-stranded spiral, like a corkscrew. It is composed of four alphabet-like bases, or nucleotides: A (adenine), T (thymine), C (cytosine), and G (guanine). A **base pair** is one of the pairs A-T or C-G.

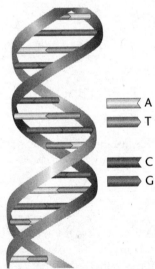

A
T

C
G

The sequence of bases in a gene code for a particular protein looks like letters in an alphabet. To make a protein, the "alphabet" base pair code of DNA is unzipped and transcribed into **RNA**, or ribonucleic acid. The bases in RNA are C, G, A, and U (uracil). U replaces T (thymine) in RNA.

The RNA is sent out of the nucleus to the **ribosomes**, where proteins are made. The letters (bases) of RNA code for **amino acids**, the building blocks of proteins.

Proteins as enzymes help cells carry out all of their important chemical reactions. For example, one **enzyme** helps a cell break down a sugar molecule in the mitochondria so it can be burned in a combustion reaction for energy.

To compare and contrast chromosomes, genes, and DNA, review their structure, function, and relationships.

The cellular process by which DNA makes proteins is shown below. The DNA triplet code is transcribed into a **codon sequence** in messenger-RNA (mRNA) in the nucleus. This new strand undergoes processing in the nucleus. The codon sequence translates into a **polypeptide**, or amino acid sequence, in the cytoplasm on the ribosome. These proteins carry out all important cell functions.

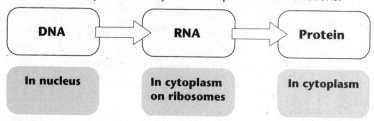

Mutations are mistakes in copying DNA. Examples of mutations that cause disorders are hemophilia and Down syndrome. A single mistake such as the one shown can cause the production of a faulty protein.

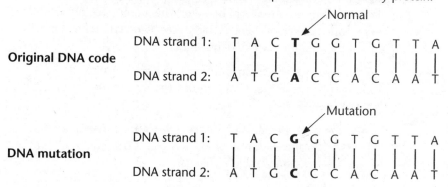

S.2.4 PROBLEM

A scientist analyzed a sample from cells and found it to contain equal amounts of cytosine, guanine, uracil, and adenine. From which part of the cell did the sample come?

(A) ribosomes

(C) chromosomes

(B) nucleus

(D) genes

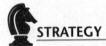STRATEGY

To answer this question, be aware of the difference between RNA and DNA.

THINK

- Remember, cytosine, guanine, uracil, and adenine are all bases for nucleic acids.

- Because uracil rather than thymine is included, the sample must be RNA rather than DNA.

- RNA is located primarily in the ribosomes, not in the nucleus. Chromosomes and genes are both part of the nucleus, so answers (B), (C), and (D) are all incorrect.

- Answer (A) is correct.

S.2.5 EXPLAIN MENDEL'S LAWS OF HEREDITY

In the mid-nineteenth century, an Austrian monk named Gregor Mendel conducted experiments on pea plants that led him to describe many of the laws of heredity. The importance of Mendel's work was not recognized until thirty years later. It remains a crucial contribution to the science of genetics.

On the TEAS Science exam, you must be able to explain the important points of Mendel's laws of heredity and the use of a Punnett square.

Review the basic elements of Mendel's work. He crossed purebred tall *(TT)* pea plants with purebred short plants *(tt)*. The result for the F1 (first) generation was all tall plants.

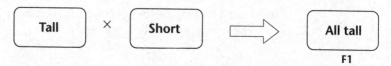

F1

Mendel explained these results by suggesting that the plants had **dominant** and **recessive** genes. In the F1 generation, all individuals had a dominant T (tall) gene, so they all had the tall **phenotype** (actual form).

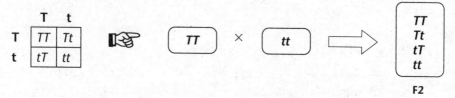

F1

Crossing the F1 generation with itself in a Tt × Tt pairing produces an F2 generation that does have short individuals. This **Punnett square** that follows shows the above cross.

Punnett Square F2

	T	t
T	*TT*	*Tt*
t	*tT*	*tt*

☞ *TT* × *tt* ⟹ *TT* *Tt* *tT* *tt*

F2

The genotypes (genetic form) and phenotypes (actual form) expected from this *Tt* × *Tt* cross would be $\frac{3}{4}$ tall and $\frac{1}{4}$ short.[‡]

Genotype: $\frac{1}{4}$ *TT*, $\frac{1}{4}$ *Tt*, $\frac{1}{4}$ *tT*, $\frac{1}{4}$ *tt*

Phenotype: $\frac{3}{4}$ tall $\frac{1}{4}$ short

For sex determination, organisms have *X* and *Y* chromosomes. An *XX* genotype creates a female; *XY* is male. A sex-linked trait such as color-blindness is carried only on X chromosomes and marked by X^c. *Y* chromosomes are "blank" for sex-linked traits—they are not **expressed**.

[‡] Fractions/percentages are approximate, as they are predicted ratios. The actual number of offspring can differ.

When a non-color-blind mother who carries the recessive color-blind X^c **allele** (X^cX) marries a normal XY father, the following genotypes result:

	X	Y
X^c	X^cX	X^cY
X	XX	XY

As you can see, the female X^cX *is not* color-blind because the X^c allele is recessive. The male X^cY *is* color-blind because the Y chromosome is not expressed for the color-blind gene.

To explain Mendel's laws of heredity, review genotypes, phenotypes, and crosses as shown in a Punnett square.

S.2.5 PROBLEM

What fraction of offspring will be short in a cross of *Tt* and *tt* parents?

(A) $\frac{1}{2}$

(C) $\frac{3}{4}$

(B) $\frac{1}{4}$

(D) all

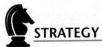

STRATEGY

To answer this question, create a Punnett square and use it to find the phenotypes.

THINK

- The Punnett square shows 2 of the 4 offspring as *tt*:

	t	*t*
T	*Tt*	*Tt*
t	*tt*	*tt*

- This means that half of the offspring will be short, making answer (A) the correct choice.

S.3 CHEMISTRY

S.3.1 RECOGNIZE BASIC ATOMIC STRUCTURE

An atom is the fundamental building block of all matter. Different elements consist of different kinds of atoms. On the TEAS Science exam, you must recognize basic atomic structure, including the subatomic particles that make up an atom. You should also review the ways in which atoms bond together by losing, gaining, or sharing electrons.

All matter is made up of **atoms**. An atom is composed of a central **nucleus** with positively charged **protons** and neutrally charged **neutrons**. Negatively charged **electrons** surround the nucleus.

Elements are composed of a single kind of atom with a particular form, mass, and structure. Each element has its own characteristic **atomic number** and **atomic mass**.

The **atomic number** tells how many protons are in the nucleus of an atom. This determines the total positive charge of the atom. It also determines the atom's chemical properties and its place in the **periodic table** of elements. Because atoms are electrically neutral, the atom must have the same number of negatively charged electrons to balance the number of protons. For example, sodium (abbreviated Na) has atomic number 11, meaning that sodium has 11 protons and 11 electrons.

Atomic mass is the number of protons plus the number of neutrons in an atom. Atomic mass is computed in **atomic mass units** (amu): 1 amu for each proton and each neutron. (Electrons have almost no mass.) Sodium's atomic mass is 11 protons + 12 neutrons = 23 amu.

The periodic table is shown on the next page. In it, atoms are arranged by atomic number (number of protons) in increasing order. The periodic table also shows atomic masses in decimal form.

To recognize basic atomic structure, review the subatomic particles that make up an atom and how its chemical properties are determined by the arrangement of its electrons.

Atoms of the same element with different numbers of neutrons are **isotopes**. For example, the most common isotope of chlorine has 17 protons + 18 neutrons = 35 amu. A rare isotope has 17 protons + 20 neutrons = 37 amu.

A **compound** is a substance composed of two or more elements, or different kinds of atoms, that are bonded together. Elements in a compound are always in fixed ratios. Sodium chloride, or table salt, is a compound.

On the atomic level, compounds are composed of molecules. Water and sugar are compounds that are composed from molecules. A water molecule is composed of hydrogen and oxygen. It is represented as H_2O; that's 2 hydrogen atoms bonded to 1 oxygen atom. A sugar (glucose) molecule is composed of 6 carbon atoms, 12 hydrogen atoms, and 6 oxygen atoms: $C_6H_{12}O_6$.

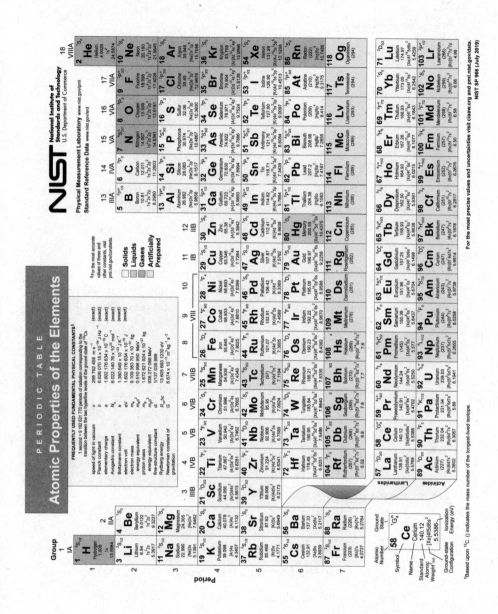

Periodic Table — Atomic Properties of the Elements (NIST SP 966, July 2019)

S.3.1 PROBLEM 1

How many neutrons does the average phosphorus atom (P) have?

(A) 15

(C) 31

(B) 16

(D) 46

STRATEGY

To answer this question, use the information on the periodic table. (Note that the atomic mass posted on the periodic table is the average mass of all isotopes for that element.)

THINK

- Remember that the number of protons (and electrons) for an element is equal to its atomic number. So phosphorus (P) has 15 protons.

- The atomic mass for P is 30.9, which rounds to 31.

- Remember that atomic mass = Protons + Neutrons. So if you write an equation for n neutrons it would be:

$$31 = 15 + n$$

- Solving for n gives $n = 16$. Phosphorus has 16 neutrons. Answer (B) is correct.

S.3.1 PROBLEM 2

Is hydrogen gas, H_2, an element or a compound?

(A) H_2 is a compound because it has 2 atoms.

(B) H_2 is an element because it has 2 atoms.

(C) H_2 is an element because it has only one kind of atom.

(D) H_2 is an element because it has two kinds of atoms.

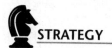

STRATEGY

Consider the definitions of both elements and compounds.

THINK

- A compound is defined as being composed of molecules having more than one kind of atom. H_2 has only one kind of atom—hydrogen—that is bonded to itself. Thus, H_2 cannot be a compound, meaning that answer (A) is incorrect.

- An element is defined as having only one kind of atom, making answer (C) the correct choice.

S.3.2 EXPLAIN CHARACTERISTIC PROPERTIES OF SUBSTANCES

Substances can be distinguished from each other by their unique properties. These include both physical and chemical properties. On the Science portion of the TEAS, you will show that you understand the characteristic properties of different substances.

All substances have both physical and chemical properties.

Physical properties can be measured without altering the essential nature of the substance. They include such properties as melting point, boiling point, freezing point, volume, viscosity, and density.

- **Melting point** is the temperature at which a substance in solid form becomes liquid.

- **Boiling point** is the temperature at which a substance in liquid form boils and turns to vapor.

- **Freezing point** is the temperature at which a substance in liquid form becomes solid. Like melting point and boiling point, freezing point is scientifically measured in units called degrees Kelvin (K).

- **Volume** measures the amount of space that a substance occupies.

- **Viscosity** measures a substance's resistance to motion when subjected to an applied force.

- **Density** measures the amount of mass a substance has per unit volume. Density is measured in units of mass or weight per volume (example: g/cm³).

Chemical properties may only be measured by altering the substance being measured. They include such properties as water-reactivity, ionization, solubility, pH (power of hydrogen), and heat of combustion.

- **Water-reactive** substances are hazardous when wet due to their chemical reaction with water.

- **Ionization energy** is the measure of the energy required to remove an electron from an atom or molecule. (First ionization energy measures removal of the most loosely held electron.) Ionization energy is measured in **joules** (also called electron volts).

- The measure of the acidity and alkalinity of a solution is called **pH**. A pH less than 7 is an acid. A pH of more than 7 is alkaline. A pH of 7 is considered neutral.

- **Heat of combustion** is the heat produced when 1 mole of a substance undergoes combustion with oxygen at constant pressure.

To explain the characteristic properties of substances, you must understand the basic physical and chemical properties such as density, melting point, and solubility.

Solubility is a chemical property that measures the ability of a substance to dissolve in a solvent. The following graph shows that solubility for sugar (glucose) increases significantly with temperature. Solubility for salt increases very slightly as temperatures rise.

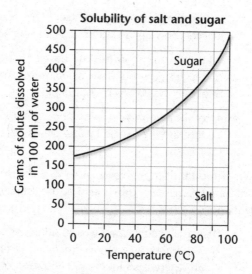

Solubility of salt and sugar

Grams of solute dissolved in 100 ml of water — Temperature (°C)

Concentration, or the amount of solute dissolved per liter, can be computed by finding the ratio of solute to solvent.

It is important to know the physical and chemical properties of **water**. A water molecule (H_2O) is asymmetrical and thus very polar. Strong attractions of hydrogen atoms for each other give water its special qualities.

- Water has a very high **heat capacity.** This is the degree to which the temperature of water changes when it gains or loses heat. In other words, water temperature tends to remain stable in response to temperature changes in the air surrounding it. It takes a significant amount of energy to boil water. A significant amount of energy must be removed for it to freeze. Water also has a high **heat of vaporization,** meaning it takes a relatively large amount of heat to vaporize.

- Water is an effective **solvent.** With its highly polar structure, water dissolves polar and ionic substances.

- The solid form of water **floats** on its liquid form. This is because ice is less dense than water. In its solid form, water's molecules, with their weak hydrogen bonds, crystallize and become rigid, maintaining separation between them.

- Water has strong **cohesion** that results in a high level of **surface tension.** Hydrogen bonds between molecules of water means that water sticks to itself. This accounts for the fact that insects can walk on water without sinking.

- Water has strong **adhesion**, based on attraction of unlike molecules. This is shown when, for example, wetting your finger allows you to pick up a pin.

- A combination of cohesion and adhesion results in **capillary action**, as when spilled water clings onto an absorbent paper towel.

Two important properties to remember are **osmosis** and **diffusion**. Both are examples of movement at the cellular level called **passive transport**.

- **Osmosis** occurs when two solutions of unequal concentration are separated by a semipermeable membrane. This generally means there is a higher concentration of water surrounding the cell than inside the cell. Water tends to move across the membrane from an area of low solute concentration to the more concentrated solution. This serves to equalize the concentrations on each side of the membrane. **Osmotic potential** refers to the tendency of water to move across a permeable membrane.

- **Diffusion** occurs when particles from an area of high concentration move spontaneously to an area of low concentration to produce a state of equilibrium.

S.3.2 PROBLEM

20 ml of olive oil weighs 18.36 g. Will an 8-g chunk of plastic that has a volume of 11 cm³ float in olive oil?

(A) Yes, because the plastic's density is greater than that of the oil.

(B) Yes, because the plastic's density is less than that of the oil.

(C) No, because the plastic's density is 0.73 g/cm³.

(D) No, because the oil's density is 0.92 g/cm³.

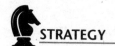

STRATEGY

To answer this question, calculate the density of both the olive oil and the piece of plastic. If the plastic has a lower density it will float.

THINK

- Olive oil density = Weight/Volume = $\frac{18.36}{20}$ = 0.92 g/cm³.
- Plastic density = Weight/Volume = $\frac{8}{11}$ = 0.73 g/cm³.
- The density of the plastic is less so it will float. Answer (B) is correct.

S.3.3 COMPARE AND CONTRAST CHANGES IN STATES OF MATTER

Ice, water, and water vapor are different states of the same substance. Differences in movement of molecules account for the different states of matter. On the TEAS exam, you must show that you understand the different states or phases of matter and be able to explain the transition from one state to another.

Every form of matter can exist in four different **states** (or phases)—**solid, liquid, gas**, and **plasma**. The focus of questions on the TEAS will be solids, liquids, and gases.

The phase of a substance is determined by the conditions of **temperature** and **pressure**.

In the graph below, water is heated to its **boiling point**—the temperature at which it changes to vapor.

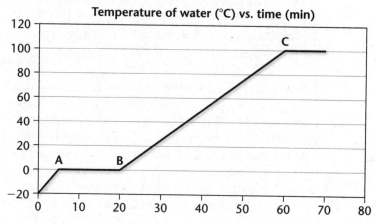

Temperature of water (°C) vs. time (min)

Heat increases the **kinetic energy** (energy of motion) of the water molecules and speeds them up. Raising the temperature to 0°C changes solid ice to liquid (point A). While heating, the icy water will remain at 0° until it completely turns to liquid (point B). Water temperature will continue to rise until it reaches 100°C, at which point it will boil (point C). The water will remain at 100° until it completely turns to a gas, or water vapor.

To compare and contrast changes in states of matter, you must be able to describe different states of matter and understand how the movement of molecules is related to these states.

In the solid phase, molecules are firmly packed in a lattice-like arrangement and held in place by atomic bonds. In the liquid phase, molecules are still relatively closely packed but have both translational and vibrational motion. In the gas phase, molecules are widely separated and move about freely at high speeds.

Changes in states of matter (or phase changes) can be **endothermic** (requiring heat) or **exothermic** (giving off heat). As a substance is heated, the molecular forces binding its molecules together are broken. The molecules begin to move away from each other.

Phase	Change	Energy
Solid to liquid	Melting	Endothermic
Liquid to gas	Vaporizing	Endothermic
Gas to liquid	Condensing	Exothermic
Liquid to solid	Freezing	Exothermic
Solid to gas	Sublimation	Endothermic
Gas to solid	Deposition	Exothermic

Changes in air pressure will change melting and boiling temperatures. For example, increasing the pressure will cause most substances to melt and boil at a temperature that is higher than normal. (Water is unusual in that increasing pressure on it when it is in solid form causes it to melt at a temperature that is *lower* than normal. This is because squeezing ice with pressure breaks up its crystal-like structure.) A phase diagram like the one that follows for water shows the different states of a substance under varying temperature and pressure.

The Three States of Matter

Vaporization occurs when liquid heats to a gas. **Condensation** is when gas cools to a liquid.

Melting occurs when a solid heats to become a liquid. **Freezing** is when a liquid cools to become a solid.

Sublimation occurs when a solid heats to become a gas. **Deposition** is when a gas cools to become a solid.

The **triple point** is the temperature and pressure at which all three states of matter can exist.

The **critical point** is the temperature and pressure at which the liquid and gas phase become identical for a pure stable substance.

S.3.3 PROBLEM

A liquid boils at 50°C. Which of the following will most likely happen if the air pressure is lowered?

(A) The liquid will boil at 55°C.

(B) The liquid will boil at 45°C.

(C) The liquid will freeze at a higher temperature than normal.

(D) The liquid will condense at a higher temperature than normal.

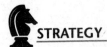

STRATEGY

To answer this question, think about how changes in air pressure affect boiling temperatures.

THINK

- Remember that decreasing pressure puts less of a "squeeze" on the substance, making it easier to boil. On the other hand, an increase in pressure squeezes matter together.

- This forces its particles to be closer together and therefore makes it harder to boil, raising the boiling temperature. Conversely, lowering the pressure makes it easier to boil the liquid, lowering the boiling temperature. Answer (B) is correct.

- Note that a lower pressure will keep particles apart and prevent them from freezing, so answer (C) is incorrect. Similarly, lower pressure will make it harder for the liquid to condense, thus lowering the temperature of condensation. That is why answer (D) is incorrect.

S.3.4 DESCRIBE CHEMICAL REACTIONS

A chemical reaction occurs when one substance changes into a new substance with a different chemical identity. Chemical reactions take place incessantly in nature as bonds between elements and compounds break down or form. On the Science portion of the TEAS exam, you must demonstrate knowledge about chemical reactions, chemical bonds, and conditions that affect them.

Chemical bonds occur when there are interactions between the electrons of two or more atoms. Molecules are groups of two or more atoms linked by chemical bonds.

Two atoms have an **ionic** bond when one or more electrons is transferred from one to the other. The atom that adds electrons has a negative charge overall. The atom that loses electrons has a positive charge overall. These atoms, with their negative or positive charges, are called **ions**. An **ionic bond** comes from the attraction of a positive ion to a negative ion. Atoms that **differ greatly** in electronegativity, such as Na (sodium) and Cl (chlorine), join to form an ionic bond. Na loses an electron to become an Na^{+1} ion. Cl gains an electron to become a Cl^- ion.

Two atoms have a **covalent** bond when they share electrons between them. Covalent bonds form between atoms with similar or identical electronegativity. When electrons are shared equally, the bond formed is **nonpolar covalent**. When electrons are shared unequally, the bond formed is **polar covalent**. In a polar covalent bond, the difference in electronegativities is not large enough to call the bond ionic.

Ionic bond

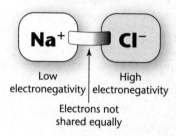

Low electronegativity | High electronegativity

Electrons not shared equally

Covalent bond

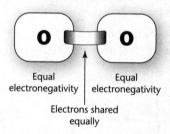

Equal electronegativity | Equal electronegativity

Electrons shared equally

To describe chemical reactions, you must be able to identify chemical bonds and explain how certain conditions and catalysts can affect chemical reactions.

Metals and nonmetals have large differences in electronegativity. Metals usually become positively charged **cations**. Nonmetals tend to become negatively charged **anions**. Ionic bonds are formed between a cation and an anion.

A **chemical reaction** occurs when chemical bonds are broken and new bonds form. In a chemical reaction, matter is never created or destroyed. This concept is referred to as the **law of conservation of matter**. Take the example of a log being burned (combustion). If you carefully weigh the log beforehand and then weigh the ash plus gases that escape afterward, you will find that they are equal.

Remember that there are five basic types of chemical reaction: **synthesis, decomposition, single replacement, double replacement,** and **combustion.**

In a **synthesis** reaction, two or more elements or compounds come together to form a single compound.

Synthesis	
Pattern	**Examples**
A + B → AB	$C + O_2 → CO_2$
	$3 H_2 + N_2 → 2 NH_3$

In a **decomposition** reaction, a single compound decomposes into two or more elements or compounds.

Decomposition	
Pattern	**Examples**
AB → A + B	$2 H_2O_2 → 2 H_2O + O_2$
	$ZnCl_2 → Zn + Cl_2$

In a **single replacement** reaction, one element switches places and replaces another element. Note that Cu and Ag switch places in the reaction below.

Single Replacement	
Pattern	**Example**
AB + C → AC + B	$Cu + 2 AgNO_3 → Cu(NO_3)_2 + 2 Ag$

In a **double replacement** reaction, two elements switch places and replace one another. Note that NO_3 and Cl switch places in the reaction below.

Double Replacement	
Pattern	**Example**
AB + CD → AD + CB	$AgNO_3 + NaCl → AgCl + NaNO_3$

In a **combustion** reaction, an organic compound combines with oxygen to produce carbon dioxide plus water. Combustion reactions are usually exothermic (giving off heat).

Combustion	
Pattern	**Example**
AB + D → AD + BD	$CH_4 + 2O_2 → CO_2 + 2H_2O$

All chemical equations for reactions must be balanced—that is, the atoms on the left side of the equation must be accounted for on the right side. For example, you can check to see whether the single replacement reaction shown below is balanced.

$$C_3H_8 + 5\,O_2 \rightarrow 3\,CO_2 + 4\,H_2O$$

Make a table to compare all atoms on the left side with all of the atoms on the right side. The table shows that the equation is balanced.

Left Side			Right Side			
C_3H_8		$5\,O_2$	$3\,CO_2$		$4\,H_2O$	
C	H	O	C	O	H	O
3 × 1	8 × 1	5 × 2	3 × 1	3 × 2	4 × 2	4 × 1
3	8	10	3	6	8	4

Remember that you must understand **acids and bases** and how they are related to **pH balance**. Common acids include HCl (hydrochloric acid), vinegar, HNO_3 (nitric acid), and H_2SO_4 (sulfuric acid). Common bases include NaOH (sodium hydroxide) and $NaHCO_3$ (sodium bicarbonate).

Acids are compounds that:

- ionize in water.
- have a sour taste.
- turn blue litmus paper red.
- have a pH less than 7.0.
- react readily with bases and many metals.
- donate H^+ ions in solution.

Bases are compounds that:

- ionize in water.
- have a bitter taste.
- turn red litmus paper blue.
- have a pH greater than 7.0.
- react readily with acids.
- donate OH^- ions in solution.

The **pH scale** measures acidity from 0 (strong acid) to 14 (strong base). Water has a pH of 7.0 and is neutral.

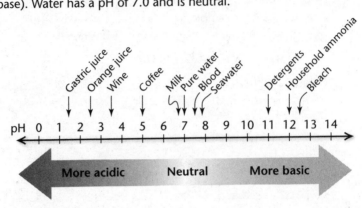

The **pH scale** is a logarithmic scale. A pH of 6.0 is 10 times as acidic as a pH of 7.0. A pH of 5.0 is 100 times as acidic as a pH of 7.0. Similarly, a pH of 9.0 is 100 times more basic than a pH of 7.0.

Litmus paper is another way to measure pH. An acidic solution turns blue litmus paper red. A base turns red litmus paper blue.

Acid–base reactions occur readily. When strong acid HCl (pH 1.0) reacts with a strong base such as NaOH (pH 13.0), it produces a salt (NaCl) and neutral water. Acids also react strongly with some metals to produce H_2 gas.

$HCl + NaOH \rightarrow NaCl + H_2O$ (Acid–base neutralization)

$Zn + 2HCl \rightarrow ZnCl_2 + H_2$ (Acid + Metal $\rightarrow H_2$)

Enzymes, or **catalysts**, are substances that speed up the rate of a biological chemical reaction but are not used up in the course of the reaction. After the reaction is complete, the enzyme remains in its same form. An enzyme lowers the amount of activation energy needed for a chemical reaction, which helps accelerate the reaction.

The substance that the enzyme acts upon is called the **substrate**. Enzymes have specific substrates. For instance, the salivary gland enzyme amylase breaks down the substrate amylose, which is starch.

Temperature and pH affect how efficient an enzyme is in catalyzing a reaction. The standard body temperature[§] is ideal for the operation of most enzymes.

S.3.4 PROBLEM

Lemon juice is about 1,000 times more acidic than coffee, which has a pH of 5. What is the pH of lemon juice?

(A) 1.0   (C) 4.0

(B) 2.0   (D) 9.0

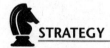

STRATEGY

To answer this question, count by powers of 10 on the pH scale.

THINK

- Remember that each unit on the logarithmic pH scale is 10 times more acidic than the previous unit.

- Since $1,000 = 10^3$, count three units back from pH 5.

- So pH 5 – 3 = pH 2. Answer (B) is correct.

S.4 SCIENTIFIC REASONING

S.4.1 IDENTIFY BASIC SCIENTIFIC MEASUREMENTS USING LABORATORY TOOLS

A nurse must be able to measure, record, and diagram data with accuracy. Scientific measurement requires a nurse to be familiar with certain tools and units. On the TEAS exam, you must demonstrate understanding of tools and measurements of volume, mass, and length.

---

§ German physician Carl Reinhold August Wunderlich first established the standard human body temperature of 98.6 degrees F in the 19th century. Modern studies, however, peg the average body temperature as somewhat lower, perhaps closer to 97.9 F, as a recent study of British patients found. There is also some variation by time of day, with the nadir generally early in the morning and the peak in the early evening.

Scientific measurement employs the metric system. This system is also called the International System of Units, or SI system (for *système internationale*—the French version of the name). This system is based on 10s, the same as decimals, so you generally need just to move the decimal point for conversion.

Metric Measurement		
Length	**Mass**	**Volume**
1,000 millimeters = 1 m	1,000 milligrams = 1 g	1,000 milliliters = 1 ℓ
100 centimeters = 1 m	100 centigrams = 1 g	100 centiliters = 1 ℓ
10 decimeters = 1 m	10 decigrams = 1 g	10 deciliters = 1 ℓ
1 meter = 1 m	1 gram = 1 g	1 liter = 1 ℓ
1 dekameter = 10 m	1 dekagram = 10 g	1 dekaliter = 10 ℓ
1 hectometer = 100 m	1 hectogram = 100 g	1 hectoliter = 100 ℓ
1 kilometer = 1,000 m	1 kilogram = 1,000 g	1 kiloliter = 1,000 ℓ

It is important to know the prefixes used in the metric system.

- Milli-   one thousandth
- Centi-   one hundredth
- Deci-   one tenth
- Deka-   ten
- Hecto-   one hundred
- Kilo-   one thousand

To identify basic scientific measurements using laboratory tools, you must be able to select the appropriate tool for different types of measurements and choose a unit of measurement suitable for what is being measured.

The base unit for **mass** is the kilogram, equal to 1,000 grams. Mass is measured using two kinds of balances.

- A **triple beam balance** includes a pan on which the object to be measured is placed; three movable-mass scales in the middle; and a balance mark on the right. When balanced, the three scales are read as follows: the middle scale shows hundreds of grams; the top scale shows tens of grams; and the bottom scale shows grams to the tenth.

- An **electronic balance** measures very small masses with great precision on a digital readout.

The base unit for **length** is the meter. Length is measured using tools such as a ruler, a tape measure, a meter stick, a gauge, and a micrometer.

The base unit for **volume of solid materials** is the cubic meter (m^3). Volume is determined by measuring an object's length, width, and height in length units and then multiplying these measurements together. A 5 cm cube has measurements of 5 cm $\times$ 5 cm $\times$ 5 cm = 125 cm^3 (volume).

The base unit for **volume of liquid** is the liter. Larger amounts of liquid volume can be measured in a volumetric flask. Small amounts are most accurately measured in a volumetric pipette. A graduated cylinder is a less precise tool for measuring liquid volume.

S.4.1 PROBLEM

Which of the following tools is used for measuring the mass of a sample?

(A) graduated cylinder

(C) triple beam balance

(B) tape measure

(D) volumetric flask

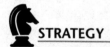 STRATEGY

Consider what type of measurement each tool is designed to make.

THINK

- Remember that mass is weight and is measured on a scale.

- A triple beam balance is a scale for measuring mass. Answer (C) is correct.

S.4.2 CRITIQUE A SCIENTIFIC EXPLANATION USING LOGIC AND EVIDENCE

Scientists perform experiments to gather data that can be analyzed. The data is used to verify or invalidate a hypothesis. On the TEAS exam, you must read data from experiments, analyze the results, and draw a valid conclusion.

Science is based on the **scientific method**. This is the method of testing an idea by designing and carrying out an experiment and then analyzing the data.

A **hypothesis** is a statement or question that can be tested. Science advances largely by the testing of hypotheses. Here are two examples of a hypothesis.

Statement form: Strength is proportional to the amount of training an athlete does.

Question form: Is strength proportional to athletic training?

For example, to test the sample hypothesis above, you need to conduct an experiment. Each group below will be tested for strength using bench press weights each week.

- **Group 1:** 90 minutes of training per day
- **Group 2:** 60 minutes of training per day
- **Group 3:** 30 minutes of training per day
- **Group 4 (Control group):** No training

The **independent variable** (input variable) in this experiment is the training time for each group. The **dependent variable** (output variable) is the number of pounds each group can bench press. The control group is exactly like the other groups except that its members will do no training.

A scientific experiment or procedure has **validity** if it is measuring the quantity or quality that is intended to be measured. Measuring a patient's temperature is a valid way to check for infection because an elevated temperature is typically associated with infections. However, measuring a patient's temperature is not a valid way to check for back pain because back pain does not typically result in an elevated temperature.

To critique a scientific explanation with logic and evidence, you must know how to collect data, analyze it, and use it to draw logical conclusions.

A scientific experiment or procedure has **reliability** if it is reproducible. This means that another person can perform the same experiment and get the same results.

A scientific experiment leads to a **conclusion** that is often expressed as a **cause-and-effect relationship**: A caused B to happen. The experimenter performs the study, collects data or evidence, analyzes it, and draws a conclusion based on cause and effect.

S.4.2 PROBLEM

A hospital manager suspects that the pay scale for nurses and the number of complaints that the hospital receives from patients are inversely proportional. The manager is organizing a study to prove her hypothesis. Which of the following would be the dependent variable for the study?

(A) number of complaints

(B) number of nurses

(C) pay scale for nurses

(D) number of patients

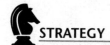

STRATEGY

Remember that to find the dependent variable, you must identify the output item that will be measured.

THINK

- The input, or independent variable, in this study is the pay scales that are given to the nurses, so answer (C) is incorrect.

- The output, or dependent variable, will emerge with each different level of pay. Answer (A) is correct.

S.4.3 EXPLAIN RELATIONSHIPS AMONG EVENTS, OBJECTS, AND PROCESSES

A nurse deals regularly with relationships of scale and cause-and-effect. It is important to identify how objects or events are related and the sequence in which things occur. On the Science portion of the TEAS, you will answer questions about relationships among events, objects, and processes.

Be sure to identify the **magnitude**—or relative size—of events and objects. Always choose the measuring unit that is scaled most appropriately to what you are measuring. The unit of measurement identifies the **scale** of what is being measured. The distance between towns, for example, should be measured in kilometers, not meters or centimeters. The size of a person's hand can be measured in centimeters. The diameter of a human hair is best measured in micrometers.

Be aware of **cause-and-effect relationships** between events, objects, and processes. For example, a smoking habit can cause a patient to have high blood pressure. Using drugs or alcohol can cause a patient to develop a dependency.

You must also explain how a **sequence** of events or processes can lead to a particular outcome. For example, overeating leads to weight gain and even obesity, which in turn can cause high blood pressure and heart disease. Be prepared to see questions about sequence and cause-and-effect relationships on the TEAS.

REMEMBER

To explain relationships among events, objects, and processes, you must be able to compare the scale of events, note the sequence of events, and identify cause-and-effect relationships between events.

S.4.3 PROBLEM

Which of the following units is suitable for measuring the weight of a powdery residue filling half of a test tube?

(A) kilograms

(B) grams

(C) milligrams

(D) micrograms

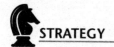

STRATEGY

Look for the measuring unit that is scaled appropriately to the thing being measured.

THINK

- The small amount of powdery residue in the test tube could best be measured in grams.

- 1 gram is 0.0022 pounds, or roughly the weight of one paper clip. Answer (B) is correct.

S.4.4 ANALYZE THE DESIGN OF A SCIENTIFIC INVESTIGATION

Scientists advance their knowledge by developing a hypothesis based on evidence, designing an investigation to test the hypothesis, and carrying out the investigation in order to affirm or reject the hypothesis. On the Science portion of the TEAS exam, you must demonstrate the ability to identify a relevant hypothesis and to analyze a scientific investigation for its strengths and weaknesses.

A hypothesis is an educated guess or insight that is relevant to the given investigation and serves as its starting point.

Each investigation must have an **independent variable, a dependent variable,** and a **control variable** or variables. The independent variable is what the experiment measures as a cause. Each experiment should have only one independent variable. If two independent variables are manipulated in the same experiment, it is impossible to be certain which is responsible for the effect. The dependent variable is what the experiment measures as an effect or outcome. The control variable is something kept constant during the experiment.

Look for strengths and weaknesses in the design of an experiment. For example, a comparison of the growth of ten pea plants under different conditions of lighting is an acceptable design. Comparing the growth of one thousand pea plants is impractical and difficult to carry out. The latter indicates a poorly designed experiment. Another weakness might be lack of a control variable, such as uniform soil conditions for the pea plants.

To analyze the design of a scientific investigation, you must be able to judge the relevance of its hypothesis, identify its variables, and point out its strengths and weaknesses.

Be ready to analyze the results of an investigation and determine whether they are valid. Look closely at the **methodology** of the experiment, or the set of procedures used to obtain the result. Think about how the experiment could have been changed or improved.

S.4.4 PROBLEM

Students are designing an investigation of waterfleas of the genus *Daphnia*. They aim to discover how changes in temperature affect the tiny crustaceans' rate of heartbeats per second. (Waterfleas are nearly transparent and their internal organs are easy to observe in live specimens.) The students plan to expose the waterfleas to temperatures from 5°C to 20°C at 5° intervals. What is the dependent variable in this experiment?

(A) temperature

(B) heartbeats/second

(C) size of the waterfleas

(D) number of waterfleas

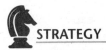

STRATEGY

Remember that the independent variable is the one that is manipulated.

THINK

- The students are exposing the waterfleas to various temperatures, so temperature is the independent variable. Answer (A) is incorrect.

- Size and number are not relevant to the experiment, so answers (C) and (D) are incorrect.

- The dependent variable is what changes in response to the independent variable. The students are measuring changes in heartbeats/second. Therefore, answer (B) is correct.

ENGLISH AND LANGUAGE USAGE

The fourth section of the TEAS covers English and Language Usage. It features 33 scored items. There are three categories of English and Language Usage objectives for the TEAS. The test items are divided among the objectives as follows.

E.1 CONVENTIONS OF STANDARD ENGLISH—12 SCORED QUESTIONS

E.1.1   Use conventions of standard English spelling.

E.1.2.   Use conventions of standard English punctuation.

E.1.3   Analyze various sentence structures.

E.2 KNOWLEDGE OF LANGUAGE—11 SCORED QUESTIONS

E.2.1   Use grammar to enhance clarity in writing.

E.2.2   Distinguish between formal and informal language.

E.2.3   Apply basic knowledge of the elements of the writing process.

E.2.4   Develop a well-organized paragraph.

E.3 USING LANGUAGE AND VOCABULARY TO EXPRESS IDEAS IN WRITING —10 SCORED QUESTIONS

E.3.1   Use context clues to determine the meaning of words or phrases.

E.3.2   Determine the meaning of words by analyzing word parts.

In addition, the TEAS English and Language Usage section features four unscored items. These items can address objectives from any of the above categories. You will have 37 minutes to complete the entire English and Language Usage section.

E.1 CONVENTIONS OF STANDARD ENGLISH

E.1.1 USE CONVENTIONS OF STANDARD ENGLISH SPELLING

Spelling can play an important part in a clinic or doctor's office. For example, a nurse or allied health professional must recognize medical homonyms—words that sound the same but are spelled differently, such as *plural* (more than one) and *pleural* (having to do with the lungs). On the English and Language Usage portion of the TEAS exam, you must be able to use the conventions of standard English spelling.

Look for homophones, or words that sound alike but are spelled differently and have different meanings. Words like *there—their—they're* are easily confused in spelling.

Remember spelling rules like *"i before e except after c or when sounded as a as in neighbor or weigh."* Be aware of exceptions to this rule, such as *caffeine* and *heir*.

Be aware of similar words that are often confused, such as *advice—advise* or *conscious—conscience*.

Use reference works such as a dictionary or thesaurus to check spelling. When using word-processing software, remember that a spell-check feature cannot catch mistakes when you type a wrong word that is spelled correctly, such as *one* instead of *ore*.

Note these examples of common homophones that often lead to spelling mistakes.

Words	Form	Sentence
it's (contraction)	it + is	It's raining outside.
its (possessive)		My car lost its pep.
who's (contraction)	who + is	Who's hungry?
whose (interrogative)		Whose shoes are these?
you're (contraction)	you + are	You're a happy dog.
your (possessive)		This is your dog.
they're (contraction)	they + are	They're eating lunch.
their (possessive)		This is their lunch.
there (adverb)		There is your lunch.

This table shows other words that are commonly confused and misspelled.

Words	Common Form	Sentence
to	preposition	I am going to the store.
too	adverb	I have too many shoes.
two	number	She has two sisters.
affect	verb	Treatment affects recovery.
effect	noun	Treatment has a major effect on recovery.
accept	verb	I accept your nomination to be president.
except	preposition	We got it all done—except the cleanup.
than	preposition	Mars is smaller than Earth.
then	adverb	The play began, and then the lights went out.
already	adverb	I already finished my homework.
all ready	adjective	The appetizers are all ready.
stationary	adjective	The fixture was stationary.
stationery	noun	He wrote me a note on his stationery.
allusion	noun	The movie included an allusion to Tarantino.
illusion	noun	Promises of quick money often turn out to be an illusion.
principle	noun	I live by a simple principle: Be nice.
principal	noun	The principal of the school was fired.
break	verb	A few items may break during the move.
brake	noun	The railroad engineer pulled the emergency brake hard to avoid an accident.
complement	noun	Crackers are the perfect complement to soup.
compliment	verb	I compliment you on your restraint.

(continued)

Words	Common Form	Sentence
advise	verb	"I advise you to remain silent," the lawyer said.
advice	noun	Megan's advice was to look for a new job.
steal	verb	Employees steal pens from work frequently.
steel	noun	The bike frame was made of super-light steel.
hear	verb	You can hear the geese flying overhead.
here	adverb	The best jobs are here in Columbus.
conscious	adjective	Evan was conscious of Al's decision to quit the firm.
conscience	noun	My conscience won't let me cheat.
device	noun	The iPad was a device that few anticipated.
devise	verb	My boss can devise a plan for saving money.
eminent	adjective	Hugh Scott is an eminent scholar.
imminent	adjective	The budget showdown is imminent.

Here are some other commonly misspelled words.

accommodate	aggravate	aging	aisle
allot	arctic	attendance	believable
believe	calendar	column	committee
conceivable	conscience	conscientious	conscious
coolly	curiosity	deceive	desirable
eligible	environment	exercise	exhaust
existence	fascinate	forfeit	grievous
government	guidance	incidentally	irresistible
library	maintenance	marriage	miniature
muscle	necessary	obedience	occasion
occurrence	persistent	possession	preference
propeller	psychiatrist	receivable	rechargeable
recommend	relieve	religious	repetition
representative	restaurant	surprise	symmetry
temperament	tendency	unnecessary	

Know the rules for forming **plurals**. The plural of a noun that ends in -*ch*, -*sh*, -*s*, -*x*, or -*z* is formed by adding -*es* instead of -*s*.

porches   sashes   bosses   sixes   buzzes

The plural of a noun that ends in a consonant and *y* is formed by replacing the -*y* with -*ies*.

hobbies   flies   allies   emergencies

The plural of a noun that ends in a vowel and *y* is formed by adding -*s*.

keys   toys   arrays

Usually, the plural of a noun that ends in a consonant and *o* is formed by adding -*es*.

tomatoes   heroes   tornadoes

The plural of a noun that ends in a vowel and *o* is usually formed by adding -*s*.

radios   portfolios   scenarios

Musical terms that end in a consonant and *o* are an exception; their plurals are formed by adding -*s*.

pianos   sopranos   tempos

The plural of a noun ending in -*f* or -*fe* is formed by replacing the *f* with *v* and adding -*es*.

wives   shelves   wolves

Letters and numbers are made plural by adding an apostrophe and -*s*.

A's   7's

Some words are irregular in the way they form plurals. You must remember the changes in their plural forms.

woman/women   person/people
mouse/mice   ox/oxen

Some words have the same form for both the singular and plural.

buffalo   deer   moose   aircraft

To use conventions of standard English spelling, learn the common spelling rules and the exceptions to those rules. Become familiar with spelling resources available online and in print.

E.1.1 PROBLEM

Which sentence is correct?

(A) Each device was rechargable, accept for the toy car.

(B) Each device was rechargeable, except for the toy car.

(C) Each devise was rechargeable, except for the toy car.

(D) Each defies was rechargeable, except for the toy car.

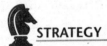

STRATEGY

Remember the conventions of standard English spelling, including common spelling rules and exceptions to the rules.

THINK

- Check each answer sentence to see if it contains a word or words that are misspelled. Check for correct use of homonyms.

- Answer (A) is incorrect because *rechargeable* is misspelled and *accept* is used for *except*.

- Answer (C) is incorrect because the verb *devise* is used instead of the noun *device*.

- Answer (D) is incorrect because the verb *defies* is used instead of the noun *device*.

- Answer (B) uses the correct spelling of the words *device*, *rechargeable,* and *except*. Therefore, (B) is the correct response.

E.1.2 USE CONVENTIONS OF STANDARD ENGLISH PUNCTUATION

Punctuation guides the reader through a text, making it easier to understand an author's meaning. Punctuation marks placed incorrectly in a sentence, however, can confuse the reader. On the TEAS exam, you must demonstrate knowledge of correct punctuation that follows the rules of standard English.

A **period** is used to end declarative sentences. Periods are also used for many abbreviations, like the following:

Dr.   etc.   Ms.   Hon.   U.S.

Periods are placed inside of quotation marks and parentheses if the parentheses enclose a full sentence. If parentheses do not enclose a full sentence, the period is placed outside of the parentheses.

We heard no barking. (The dog was asleep.)

The recipe called for lots of healthy ingredients (and butter and sugar).

Commas are used in a variety of situations following these general rules:

- **Series of three or more:** Use commas to separate items. This is actually optional, but is generally preferred.

   The patient had no money, identification, or insurance.

   We are improving our performance with respect to response time for patients, overall hospital infection rate, and family-patient interaction satisfaction.

- **After an introductory word group:** Use commas after phrases or clauses that come before the subject.

   In addition to all her other accomplishments, Marta was the first one in her family to attend college.

   Although Gwen was the first one in her family to attend college, her parents made sure each of her younger sisters did too.

- **Before a coordinating conjunction** *(and, so, but, for, or, nor, yet):* Use a comma along with a coordinating conjunction to connect independent clauses.

Tupac Shakur was clearly a troubled individual, but he was also surely a hip-hop genius.

Beyoncé was worried that something would go wrong, so she lip-synched her performance during the Super Bowl.

- **To mark interruptions within a sentence:** Use two commas to set off the interruption.

    The Dallas Cowboys, though widely despised, are also perhaps the most popular team in the NFL.

Use an **apostrophe** in the following ways:

- **To show letters that have been left out in a contraction:**

don't	you're	I'm	isn't
he's	hasn't	won't	doesn't
can't	we're	I'll	we've
you've	it's	who's	they're

When you use conventions of standard English punctuation, you employ punctuation marks to clarify meaning, set off quotations or parenthetical material, and indicate possession or conjunctions.

Note these tricky examples of apostrophe usage that often cause mistakes.

	Form	Sentence
it's (contraction)	it + is	It's raining outside.
its (possessive)		My car lost its pep.
who's (contraction)	who + is	Who's hungry?
whose (interrogative)		Whose shoes are these?
you're (contraction)	you + are	You're a happy dog.
your (possessive)		This is your dog.
they're (contraction)	they + are	They're eating lunch.
their (possessive)		This is their lunch.
there (adverb)		There is your lunch.

- **To show possession:**

  Hal's bicycle   Lina's job   Francis's district

  Adam and Franco's restaurant (belongs to both)

  the members' decision (decision of more than one member)

  the United States' legacy

- **Possessive pronouns do not take apostrophes.**

  yours   ours   theirs   its

- **In acronyms and other unusual forms, use apostrophes only when necessary to avoid confusion.**

  1980s   PDFs   URLs

  do's and don'ts   p's and q's

Use **quotation marks** to identify a person's exact words.

Bonnie said, "Where have all the flowers gone?"

"My friend Marcus is a whiz with tools," Sally told us.

"Only five districts have voted!" Karl cried.

"The die is cast," Churchill lamented, "and it looks like there will be war."

Use quotation marks to set off titles of songs, poems, and articles (but not book titles or titles of larger works or publications):

The Beatles' song "Taxman" on the album *Revolver*

Robert Frost's poem "The Road Not Taken" in *Great American Poems*

The article "Stocks Rise for the Week" in *The Wall Street Journal*

Use a **colon** to introduce a list, an extended quotation, an example, or a conclusion.

Todd instructed me to purchase these items: bread, flour, yeast, cinnamon, sugar, and milk. (list)

John F. Kennedy famously stated: "Ask not what your country can do for you. Ask what you can do for your country." (extended quotation)

Brad had one big thing working against him: his rather abrasive personality. (example)

The obesity data made one thing clear: Drinking soda is not good for you. (conclusion)

Use a **semicolon** with conjunctive adverbs such as *however, still, thus, nevertheless,* and *therefore* to separate independent clauses.

A small 1 percent of the population pays almost 40 percent of all federal taxes; however, this segment also owns a sizable percentage of the nation's wealth.

Use a semicolon to separate listed items that also include commas.

I've applied to the University of Wisconsin in Madison, Wisconsin; the University of Oklahoma in Norman, Oklahoma; the University of North Carolina in Greensboro, North Carolina; and Harvard University in Cambridge, Massachusetts.

Use a **hyphen** to combine two words to create a compound modifier.

Nora's last-second shot tied the score.

Use a **dash** to set off an important fact or amplification of a fact.

The legendary 396-cubic-inch Chevrolet engine—which got less than 16 miles per gallon—was symbolic of a time when gasoline was cheap and environmental concerns were nonexistent.

Use **parentheses** to set off nonessential or explanatory words.

Elvis Costello (real name: Declan Patrick McManus) has proved to be one of the most versatile and imaginative songwriters of his generation.

E.1.2 PROBLEM

Which sentence is punctuated correctly?

(A) Dave, an insightful and talented therapist, is nevertheless prone to jumping to conclusions.

(B) Dave is an insightful and talented therapist but, he is nevertheless prone to jumping to conclusions.

(C) Although Dave, is an insightful and talented therapist, he is nevertheless prone to jumping to conclusions.

(D) Dave an insightful and talented therapist, is nevertheless prone to jumping to conclusions.

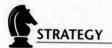 **STRATEGY**

Use the rules of standard English punctuation to evaluate the sentences.

THINK

- Answer (B) fails to precede the coordinating conjunction *but* with a comma, so it is incorrect.

- Answer (C) incorrectly places a comma between *Dave* and *is,* the subject and verb in the introductory dependent clause.

- Answer (D) does not place a comma after *Dave* to separate it from the appositive phrase *an insightful and talented therapist,* so it is incorrect.

- Answer (A) sets off the appositive properly. Therefore, (A) is correct.

E.1.3 ANALYZE VARIOUS SENTENCE STRUCTURES

A sentence can be built in many different ways. It can be simple, with only the most basic parts, or incredibly complex. By analyzing sentence structure, you can see how an author puts together a sentence to create meaning. On the English and Language Usage portion of the TEAS exam, you must demonstrate knowledge of sentence structure and the parts that make up a sentence.

- To analyze the structure of a sentence, identify its pattern: simple, compound, complex, or compound-complex.

- Identify clauses and phrases and see how they are combined in the sentence.

- Identify the eight parts of speech—noun, pronoun, verb, adjective, adverb, preposition, conjunction, and interjection—and see which ones are used in the sentence and how they are used.

- Diagram the sentence to show how the various parts fit together.

There are **four types of sentences:** declarative (a statement), imperative (a command), interrogative (a question), and exclamatory (an exclamation or emotional statement).

The **four sentence patterns** are as follows:

Simple: Contains only a subject and predicate.

The inquisitive kitten crept up to the stuffed animal on the floor.

The simple subject is the noun *kitten,* and the simple predicate is the verb *crept.* The complete subject is *The inquisitive kitten.* The complete predicate is *crept up to the stuffed animal on the floor.*

Compound: Contains two independent clauses joined by a coordinating conjunction. A good mnemonic device for coordinating conjunctions is FANBOYS (**f**or, **a**nd, **n**or, **b**ut, **o**r, **y**et, **s**o).

The home team played well, but the visitors prevailed in the end.

The home team played well is one independent clause, and *the visitors prevailed in the end* is another independent clause. The two clauses are connected by the coordinating conjunction *but.*

Complex: Contains an independent clause and a (dependent) subordinate clause.

Since her art students are studying impressionism, Ms. Watanabe took them on a field trip to an exhibit of Monet paintings at the local museum.

The independent clause in this sentence is *Ms. Watanabe took them on a field trip to an exhibit of Monet paintings at the local museum.* The dependent subordinate clause is *Since her art students are studying impressionism.*

Compound-Complex: Contains two independent clauses and a dependent (subordinate) clause.

Although Ebony had sold several of her paintings, she apparently lost the desire to paint, for she concentrated instead on her gardening business.

The two independent clauses in this sentence are *she apparently lost the desire to paint* and *she concentrated instead on her gardening business.* The dependent subordinate clause is *Although Ebony had sold several of her paintings.*

To analyze various sentence structures, become familiar with the eight parts of speech and the four main sentence patterns. Identify clauses and phrases. Practice with sentence structure by diagramming sentences.

As you analyze sentences, it is important to recognize **clauses and phrases**. A clause has both a subject and a verb. A phrase may lack one or both of these. A phrase is a group of words (usually part of a clause) that form a conceptual unit. Look at the sentence below.

When Bethany grabbed the steering wheel, the boat began to veer wildly in every direction.

When Bethany grabbed the steering wheel is a dependent clause, and *the boat began to veer wildly in every direction* is an independent clause. The phrase *in every direction* is a prepositional phrase.

The eight parts of speech are as follows:

Noun: a word for a person, place, thing, or idea.

Frank believed in *America, democracy,* and the *ballot box.*

Verb: a word that shows action or a state of being.

The dog *barked* and *howled,* but Hannah *was* so tired that she *did* not *awaken.*

Pronoun: a word that takes the place of a noun. Here the pronoun *she* refers to the noun *Maude.*

Maude read the newspaper while *she* ate breakfast.

Adjective: a word that modifies a noun or pronoun.

I got the *red* scissors from the *bureau* drawer to clip the *beautiful* photo.

Adverb: a word that modifies a verb, an adjective, or another adverb. Here the adverb *very* modifies the adverb *carefully;* the adverb *carefully* modifies the verb *lifted;* and the adverb *bright* modifies the adjective *yellow.*

Walter *very carefully* lifted the lid off the *bright* yellow coffee cup.

Preposition: a word that defines the relationship between other words and phrases in a sentence.

Dakota walked *around* the block and *into* the restaurant.

Conjunction: a word that joins together words, phrases, or clauses.

Zooey *and* Sim arrived late, *but* we still had a great time with them.

Interjection: a word, phrase, or short clause that expresses strong emotion.

Rats! The Broncos beat my favorite team in the Super Bowl.

To see how sentence parts fit together, it helps to **diagram a sentence**. Compare this sentence to its diagram below.

The timbers of the ancient ship groaned and creaked in the rising waves.

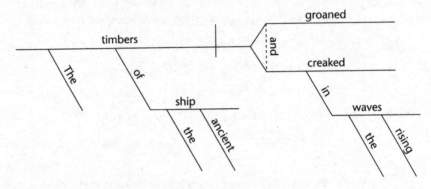

E.1.3 PROBLEM

Which of the following statements about this sentence is true?

Although Senator Simpson is now obsessed with budgetary deficits, when he was in power, he saw nothing wrong with running a large deficit.

(A) *Although Senator Simpson is now obsessed with budgetary deficits* is an independent clause.

(B) *Although Senator Simpson is now obsessed with budgetary deficits* is a dependent clause.

(C) *When he was in power* is an independent clause.

(D) *He saw nothing wrong with running a large deficit* is a dependent clause.

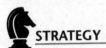

STRATEGY

Use your knowledge about the four main sentence structures and the difference between independent and dependent clauses.

THINK

- An independent clause must be able to stand on its own as a sentence. *Although Senator Simpson is now obsessed with budgetary deficits* and *When he was in power* cannot stand on their own, so neither clause is independent. Answers (A) and (C) are incorrect.

- *He saw nothing wrong with running a large deficit* can stand on its own, so it is independent, not dependent. Answer (D) is incorrect.

- As already stated, *Although Senator Simpson is now obsessed with budgetary deficits* cannot stand on its own, so it is a dependent clause. Answer (B) is correct.

E.2 KNOWLEDGE OF LANGUAGE

E.2.1 USE GRAMMAR TO ENHANCE CLARITY IN WRITING

Good grammar and thoughtful word choice are tools a writer uses to create sentences with precision. They enable a writer to deliver a message with force and clarity. On the TEAS exam, you must demonstrate how to use grammar to write with greater clarity.

- Look for complete sentences in a piece of writing. Make sure there are no run-on sentences or sentence fragments.

- Make sure past, present, and future tense are used consistently throughout.

- Look for subject-verb agreement and pronoun-antecedent agreement.

- Look for transition words that connect ideas and clarify their relationship for the reader.

- Look for examples of ambiguous language and replace it with precise wording.

- Choose words that express the exact shade of meaning you intend to convey.

Avoid **run-on sentences, sentences with a comma splice**, and **sentence fragments.**

> Questions remain about the budget the mayor has raised several concerns.
> (Run-on sentence: Two independent clauses are incorrectly joined with no punctuation.)

> Transportation presents a number of problems, a new railway is being planned.
> (Comma splice: Two independent clauses are incorrectly joined with a comma.)

> The city council, by addressing this issue.
> (Sentence fragment: The sentence is incorrect because it lacks a predicate.)

Subject and verbs should always agree in number. A singular subject requires a singular verb. A plural subject requires a plural verb.

> The *player runs* laps around the field after practice.
> (The singular subject, *player,* takes a singular verb, *laps.*)

> The *players run* laps around the field after practice.
> (The plural subject, *players,* takes a plural verb, *run.*)

Pronouns and antecedents should always agree. Subjective personal pronouns include *I, you, he, she, we,* and *they.* Objective personal pronouns include *me, you, him, us, her,* and *them.*

> *He* and Laurie both graduated the same year.
> (*He,* a subjective pronoun, is used as a subject.)

> The doctor gave a compliment to Meryl and *me.*
> (*Me,* an objective pronoun, is used as an object.)

To use grammar to enhance clarity in writing, focus on wording that is precise, not ambiguous, and follow grammar rules consistently.

The use of **tense** (past, present, future) should be consistent throughout.

> **Incorrect:** The mayor *gave* a speech that *will describe* his plan to fight poverty.
> (Past tense verb *gave* is used with future tense *will describe*.)

> **Correct:** The mayor *gave* a speech that *described* his plan to fight poverty.
> (Past tense verb *gave* is used with past tense *described*.)

Transition words signal a connection between ideas.

> Jazz bandleader Duke Ellington brought a new sophistication to jazz composition. *Moreover,* he maintained this high standard for decades.
> (*Moreover* indicates the information is added to that of the first sentence.)

> Louis Armstrong was born into a bleak setting of poverty and crime in New Orleans. *Nonetheless,* he rose to become one of the greatest jazz instrumentalists in history.
> (*Nonetheless* indicates Armstrong rose despite his humble origins.)

Vague and ambiguous language should be replaced with precise wording.

> **Vague:** The stuff they say on TV is hard to believe.
> **Better:** The claims made for certain products on TV commercials are wildly exaggerated.

> **Ambiguous:** Visiting relatives can make a person weary and irritable.
> (Are the relatives visiting or is the person visiting the relatives?)
> **Better:** Visiting one's relatives can be wearisome and irritating.

Word choices should be made carefully to get the proper shade of meaning.

> Our halfback *darted* into the end zone as time expired.
> (*Darted* indicates moving rapidly in a straight line.)

> Our halfback *strolled* into the end zone as time expired.
> (*Strolled* indicates moving with ease and confidence.)

> Our halfback *dodged* into the end zone as time expired.
> (*Dodged* indicates moving to avoid tacklers in a swarm.)

E.2.1 PROBLEM

Which sentence is correct?

(A) Both Eric and me ask that you give him and me your support.

(B) Both Eric and me ask that you give he and I your support.

(C) Both Eric and I ask that you give him and I your support.

(D) Both Eric and I ask that you give him and me your support.

STRATEGY

Use your knowledge about correct use of subjective and objective pronouns.

THINK

- Check to see that the correct subjective and objective pronouns are used.

- The subjective *Eric and I* must be used as the subject of the sentence, not the objective *Eric and me,* so answer (A) and answer (B) are both incorrect.

- The objective form *him and me* must be used as indirect object. Therefore, answer (C) is incorrect.

- In answer (D), the correct forms of the pronouns are used. The correct response is answer (D).

E.2.2 DISTINGUISH BETWEEN FORMAL AND INFORMAL LANGUAGE

Authors write in a style that is suited to their intended audience. For example, a historian might write in a formal style for a professional journal and in a more relaxed style for a book aimed at general readers. A student writes differently for a book report than what's appropriate in a text message to a friend. On the TEAS exam, you must distinguish between formal and informal language and evaluate which is appropriate for the intended audience.

First, determine the purpose and audience for a piece of writing. Next, decide whether the author's style is appropriate for that purpose and audience. Finally, identify examples of formal language or informal language (slang, colloquialisms, etc.).

A writer's style is accomplished through tone, diction, and word choice. One way to think of style is as the voice of the writer. Look at the difference in style of the two examples below.

Formal: Claudia was aware that pizza is excessively high in fat and calories.

Informal: Claudia was like, pizza is so fattening, you know?

A formal style is appropriate for a public speech, research report, scholarly article, business letter, or historical essay. Readers expect these modes of writing to have correct diction, a formal tone, and precise word choices. The author can use more sophisticated syntax to achieve the desired shades of meaning.

In evaluating formal and informal language, see if the style of writing is appropriate for the genre and intended audience.

An informal style is more appropriate for casual writing or entertainment purposes, such as a comical essay, a blog post, or a personal letter. The tone of this mode of writing is usually light and breezy. Often the writer will address the reader in the second person, as *you*. Look at these two examples of how to treat a science topic.

Formal: This week presents an excellent opportunity to view the Orionid meteor shower, the second of two spectacular showers that take place each year due to our planet passing through dust emitted by Halley's Comet.

Informal: With Earth whooshing through the tail of old Halley's Comet, you're about to get one whale of a nighttime show meteor-wise.

Authors also vary their style with slang, colloquial expressions, and idioms. These elements can help a writer establish a bond with the reader by using casual, everyday language that expresses honesty or a "down-home" feel.

Slang is informal language that is nonstandard and usually not appropriate in formal writing. It includes the trendy words of the day, with recent examples including the verb *ghost* (to abruptly cut off all communication with), *salty* (upset or angry), *tea* (gossip), *chill* (relax), *lit* (cool), *crib* (home), and *GOAT* (greatest of all time). Certain professions have their own slang, or **jargon**. Musicians might employ the words *gig* (show) and *jam* (play with other musicians). A basketball player might refer to a *dime* (a pass leading to a made basket), a *brick* (an off-target shot), an *alley-oop* (a pass for a dunk), or a *buzzer beater* (a successful last-second shot).

Colloquialisms are expressions or figures of speech that are associated with a region and/or time period. Instead of a soft drink, a person in New York might drink a *soda*, while a Midwesterner would have a *pop*. During World War II, a dancer might have *cut a rug*, while in the 1980s he or she might have *boogied down*.

Idioms are colloquial metaphors, such as the following.

raining cats and dogs	(raining hard)
hit the hay	(go to bed)
paint the town red	(have a wild night out)
a piece of cake	(easy to do)
a drop in the bucket	(an action with little overall effect)

E.2.2 PROBLEM

Read the passage. Then answer the question.

In Shakespeare's play *Hamlet,* the title character confronts a situation that seemingly leaves him paralyzed and unable to act decisively. At night on the battlements of Elsinore Castle, Hamlet is visited by his father's ghost, one of literature's great spirits with an axe to grind. The ghost solemnly explains how he was murdered by his own brother, the man who now sits on his throne, wears his crown, and has married his widow. Hamlet is charged by his father's spirit with the awesome task of bloody revenge.

Which of the following is not appropriate to the overall tone of this passage?

(A) seemingly leaves him paralyzed

(B) At night, on the battlements of Elsinore

(C) with an axe to grind

(D) with the awesome task of bloody revenge

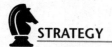

STRATEGY

Refer to the rules about the use of formal and informal language.

THINK

- Note that this piece of writing is a formal literary essay on *Hamlet*. Thus, the tone and diction should be formal throughout.

- The colloquial expression *with an axe to grind,* meaning "to have a grievance against someone," is more suitable to informal writing. Answer (C) is correct.

E.2.3 APPLY BASIC KNOWLEDGE OF THE ELEMENTS OF THE WRITING PROCESS

The writing process includes each step of creating a piece of writing, from planning to final revision. Every writer has her or his own approach to the writing process. The procedure may change according to what kind of writing is required for a project. The steps involved in prewriting, writing, and revision often blend into each other as the writer proceeds. On the English and Language Usage section of the TEAS exam, you will demonstrate knowledge of the basic writing process.

In the **prewriting stage**, you should do everything necessary to prepare to write. This can include making a schedule for writing, deciding on a plan or purpose for writing, brainstorming ideas about the topic, doing research about the topic, and making an outline to organize your research.

In the **writing stage**, you should draft the piece of writing and compile the sources you need as references. A draft is a version of a piece of writing that is unfinished.

In the **revision stage**, you should check your draft to see that the material is organized properly and to edit your writing for clarity. You should also look for errors in grammar and punctuation.

Prewriting (planning/preparation/outline)

Decide on a topic and focus the topic into a thesis statement. Think about your audience for this piece of writing. Try to write a thesis statement that will capture the reader's interest.

Topic: The U.S. National Park System

Thesis Statement: Creating a national park system was a radical idea that sought to give all Americans the chance to enjoy their country's natural beauty.

After researching the topic, you might create an outline to organize your information.

I. The Beginnings of a U.S. National Park System

    A. Discovery of Yosemite in 1851

    B. Expeditions to Yosemite by James Mason Hutchings and others

    C. Congress sets aside Yosemite as a park to be administered by California

    D. Yosemite becomes a national park in 1890

II. Establishing the U.S. National Park System

    A. President Grant signs the bill creating Yellowstone Park, the first national park

        a. Yellowstone stretches over 2 million acres

        b. Attendance increased five-fold in the first year

    B. Sequoia National Park and General Grant National Park are also created

    C. In 1916 President Woodrow Wilson signs the act for the National Park Service

Writing (drafting/compiling sources)

Use your research notes and outline to draft your essay. Follow the plan in your outline to organize your essay. Concentrate on creating a strong opening that introduces the topic and a strong closing that sums up your research. You might adapt your thesis statement to create your topic sentence in the first paragraph.

Compile your sources into the proper format for a bibliography, or list of sources. Make sure you identify sources used for direct quotes.

Jen A. Huntley, *The Making of Yosemite: James Mason Hutchings and the Origin of America's Most Popular Park,* University of Kansas Press, 2011.

Revision (organization/clarity/grammar)

Check your draft for its organization. See if a sentence or section works better in another location. For example, you might decide that the description of how Yosemite became a national park in 1890 (item D in Section I) would be more appropriate if moved between items A and B in Section II, on Establishing the U.S. National Park System.

Next, reread your draft carefully to see if certain words, phrases, or sentences need to be rewritten for clarity. You should also check for any errors in grammar or punctuation.

To apply the elements of the writing process, demonstrate knowledge of prewriting, writing, and revision.

E.2.3 PROBLEM

Creating a focused thesis statement should be done in which stage of the writing process?

(A) Prewriting

(C) Writing

(B) Prewriting or Revision

(D) Revision

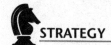

STRATEGY

Think about what happens at each stage of the writing process.

THINK

- A focused thesis statement helps direct a writer's research on a topic.

- The thesis statement must be created at the first stage of the writing process, which is Prewriting. Answer (A) is correct.

E.2.4 DEVELOP A WELL-ORGANIZED PARAGRAPH

Paragraphs are the building blocks of a piece of writing. Each paragraph adds an important idea to the overall topic. A paragraph can be short and punchy or long and very detailed. It is important that each paragraph be organized logically and written with clarity and focus. On the English and Language Usage section of the TEAS exam, you must demonstrate knowledge of how to develop a well-organized paragraph.

- First, write a topic sentence that sets out the idea you intend to explore in the paragraph.

- Next, add supporting details that provide more information about the topic sentence. Check to see that all the details belong in the paragraph.

- Finally, end the paragraph with a conclusion or transition. A good concluding sentence either wraps up the main idea in the paragraph or connects it to an important idea in the following paragraph.

Notice how this writer created a well-organized paragraph on the tennis-playing sisters Venus and Serena Williams.

The **topic sentence** presents the main idea of the paragraph:

In discussing athletes who revolutionized their sport, one can't ignore the Williams sisters, Venus and Serena, who brought a new aggressiveness and athletic style to professional tennis.

Supporting details add important information to the topic sentence. The facts should be organized and presented logically. They might be written in time order, in order of importance, according to cause and effect, or by some other pattern. The supporting details below are arranged in chronological order.

Growing up in the tough neighborhoods of Compton in Los Angeles, Venus and Serena learned to play tennis on the public courts. In 2000, Venus electrified the tennis world by winning the singles title at both Wimbledon and the U.S. Open. Two years later, Serena defeated Venus in the Wimbledon final and replaced her as the world's top-ranked player.

A concluding or transition sentence sums up the main idea of the paragraph or connects it to the next paragraph. The sentence below is a transition to the following paragraph.

Longtime tennis fans marveled at the Williams sisters' early success, but Venus and Serena were just getting started.

To write a well-organized paragraph, see that you have a topic sentence, supporting details, and a strong conclusion or clear transition to the next paragraph. Make sure there are no unnecessary details in the paragraph.

E.2.4 PROBLEM

Read the following topic sentence. Then answer the question.

The 2010 explosion of the Deepwater Horizon offshore drilling rig sent millions of gallons of oil pouring into the Gulf of Mexico, presenting engineers with an enormous clean-up problem.

Which of the following would be the best supporting detail for a paragraph organized by problem/solution?

(A) There were several reasons why the Deepwater Horizon oil spill threatened to become one of the worst environmental disasters in history.

(B) One method for dealing with the disaster involved dumping chemicals into the ocean to break up the heavy oil much like dishwashing detergents dissolve grease.

(C) Immediately experts began to debate about who was most responsible for the environmental catastrophe.

(D) Experts warned that the spill would have a major impact on the environment in the Gulf area, including wildlife and vegetation.

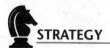

STRATEGY

Use your knowledge about how to organize a paragraph logically.

THINK

- The correct answer should be a sentence that provides a possible solution to the problem presented in the topic sentence.

- Answer (A) is incorrect because it introduces reasons why the oil spill threatened to be so serious, but not possible solutions to the problem.

- Answer (C) focuses on the debate about who was most responsible, so it is incorrect.

- Answer (D) focuses on a cause-and-effect organization, so it is incorrect.

- Answer (B) presents a method for dealing with the disaster, which is a possible solution to the problem. Answer (B) is correct.

E.3 USING LANGUAGE AND VOCABULARY TO EXPRESS IDEAS IN WRITING

E.3.1 USE CONTEXT CLUES TO DETERMINE THE MEANING OF WORDS OR PHRASES

Context clues are hints to the meaning of a word or phrase that are found in the surrounding text. They include synonyms and antonyms, explanatory words or definitions, and words that establish a tone that hints at the correct meaning. On the TEAS exam, you will use context clues to determine the meaning of words or phrases.

When you encounter an unfamiliar word, examine how it is used in the sentence. Think about what part of speech it is. See if there is a definition or explanation of the word in the surrounding text.

Look for synonyms or antonyms of the unfamiliar word. These can lead you to guess the meaning.

Think about the mood or tone of the sentence or passage in which the unfamiliar word appears. What is the overall mood of the sentence? Is the word used sarcastically or humorously?

When you encounter an unfamiliar phrase, decide if it is an idiom. This is a phrase in which the actual meaning is different from the literal meaning of the individual words, as in *hold your tongue*.

To use context clues to determine meaning, look at the words surrounding the unfamiliar word or phrase, think of synonyms for words with multiple meanings, and note the mood or tone of the passage.

Types of Context Clues

Definition: Political prisoners in the old Soviet Union were sent to the *gulag*, a network of prison camps in the arctic north.

> The word *gulag* is followed by the definition *a network of prison camps in the arctic north.*

Synonym: Her success on the pop charts was *transitory*, a fleeting moment that she would never experience again.

> The word *fleeting* has a very similar meaning to *transitory*—something that does not last.

Antonym: The crowd's *raucous* antics contrasted sharply with their usual subdued behavior.

> The word *subdued* is contrasted with *raucous* as its opposite or antonym.

Choose from among multiple meanings: The *break* the investigators were seeking came as they were discussing the case during their *break*.

> The first *break* means an "opening or breakthrough," while the second *break* means "a pause during the workday."

Mood or tone: *Jubilation* overtook the crowd as the band struck up a lively tune and an abundance of colorful balloons filled the sky.

> The details of the sentence (the band playing a lively tune, the balloons filling the sky) indicate that *jubilation* means "joyfulness."

Idiom: I tried to keep the surprise party for Jaden a secret, but Harvey slipped up and *let the cat out of the bag*.

> The context clues indicate that the idiom *let the cat out of the bag* means "to reveal a secret."

E.3.1 PROBLEM

Read the following sentence. Then answer the question.

> The sight of his broken coffee mug *incensed* Mr. Sacks, but we soon managed to pacify him by explaining it was an accident.

Which of the following words is an antonym that provides a clue to the meaning of *incensed*?

(A) broken

(C) explaining

(B) pacify

(D) accident

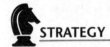

STRATEGY

Use context clues to analyze the meaning of words in a sentence.

THINK

- Context clues can include synonyms or antonyms of an unfamiliar word.

- The word *pacify* is an antonym of the word *incensed*. Mr. Sacks is incensed, or very angry, about his broken mug, but then calms down when he learns the explanation. Answer (B) is correct.

E.3.2 DETERMINE THE MEANING OF WORDS BY ANALYZING WORD PARTS

Sometimes you can figure out the meaning of a word by examining its parts. Prefixes and suffixes change the meaning of a word's stem or root. Knowing how affixes alter a root word's meaning is especially helpful for healthcare professionals dealing with a medical term like *hypoglycemic*. (The prefix *hypo-* means "low"; *hypoglycemic* means "low blood sugar levels.") On the TEAS exam, you must demonstrate the ability to find the meaning of words—especially medical terms—by analyzing their word parts.

- Analyze an unfamiliar word to identify its root.

- Determine if the word contains a prefix or suffix. A prefix is added to the beginning of a root word to change its meaning. A suffix is added to the end of a word to change its meaning.

- Figure out the meaning of the word by combining the meanings of the root and the prefix and/or suffix.

Find lists of prefixes and suffixes in books on English usage or on the internet. Here is a chart of words related to the medical field with roots and prefixes or suffixes.

Prefix	Root	Word	Meaning
a- (not)	rhythm	arrhythmia	irregular heartbeat
endo- (inside)	scope	endoscope	an instrument to look inside the body
hyper- (excessive)	tension	hypertension	high blood pressure
pre- (before)	natal	prenatal	before birth
post- (after)	operative	postoperative	period following surgery
Suffix	Root	Word	Meaning
-ectomy (removal)	appendix	appendectomy	removal of the appendix
-emia (blood condition)	septic	septicemia	bloodstream infection
-itis (inflammation)	colon	colitis	inflammation of the inner lining of the colon
-ology (study)	psyche	psychology	study of the human mind and behavior

To determine the meaning of words by analyzing word parts, look for prefixes or suffixes that modify the meaning of the root.

E.3.2 PROBLEM

Which prefix could be added to the word *cover* to form a word with the opposite meaning?

(A) anti-

(B) dis-

(C) re-

(D) un-

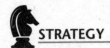

STRATEGY

Use your knowledge about how prefixes and suffixes change the meaning of a root word.

THINK

- Think about the meaning of each word formed by adding the prefix to the word *cover*. To *cover* is to protect or conceal something.

- Answer (A) is incorrect because *anticover* is not a word.

- Answer (B) is incorrect because *discover* means "to find something," which is not quite the opposite meaning of *cover*.

- Answer (C) is incorrect because *recover* means "to get something back or recuperate," neither of which is the opposite meaning of *cover*.

- The word *uncover* means "to remove the cover or reveal something," which is the opposite meaning of *cover*. Answer (D) is correct.

Glossary

absolute value: A bracket function that turns any value within its brackets positive; for example, $|3-5| = |-2| = 2$

acid: A sour, corrosive chemical that ionizes in water to form H^+ ions and has a pH of below 7.0

adjective: A word that modifies a noun or pronoun; for example, a *red* coat, a *small* dog

advance directive: A legal document that ensures that medical choices are made according to the patient's wishes when the patient is unable to make them

adverb: A word that modifies a verb, adjective, or another adverb; for example, Jane is *very* smart. Jane walks *slowly*.

allele: A form of a gene that codes for proteins that produce given traits; for example, Mendel's peas had a dominant *tall* allele and a recessive *short* allele

amino acid: One of 20 small nitrogen-containing organic acids that serve as building blocks for all proteins

antecedent: In grammar, the noun to which a pronoun refers; for example, in the sentence, "Charles wants Sue to look at him," *Charles* is the antecedent of *him*.

antibody: A blood protein that is made by B cells to bind to foreign antigens that enter the body so they can be eliminated

antigen: A toxin or foreign substance that produces an immune response in the body; for example, the immune response might be the production of antibodies

antonym: A word that has the opposite meaning of another word

apostrophe: A punctuation mark (') that shows ownership or identifies missing letters in contractions; for example, *Larry's* book, or *isn't*

area: What is enclosed within the perimeter of a figure, expressed in square units

artery: A blood vessel that carries blood *away* from the heart

atom: The fundamental unit of matter that makes up the 118 different elements, or forms of matter; an atom consists of a central nucleus containing protons, neutrons, and outer electrons

atomic mass: The mass of a single atom, usually expressed in atomic mass units (amu)

atomic number: The number that identifies a particular element on the periodic table; it tells how many protons and electrons that atom has; for example, carbon, with atomic number 6, has 6 protons and 6 electrons

atomic radius: The distance from an atom's nucleus to its outermost electron

atrium: One of the top chambers of the heart that receives blood from the body

author's purpose: The aim of the author in writing the text; typically to explain, persuade, entertain, or express feelings

axon: The long, thin, conductive part of the neuron that conducts impulses away from the neuron cell body

B cells: A type of white blood cell that produces antibodies

bacteria: one-celled germs that are able to multiply quickly; bacteria exist nearly everywhere on Earth and are essential to the planet's ecosystems.

base: A chemical that produces OH^{-1} ions in solution, has a pH of greater than 7.0, and reacts with acids

bases: One of the four "alphabet letters" that make up the genetic code for DNA: A (adenine), T (thymine), C (cytosine), and G (guanine)

bias: A prejudice that is typically based on a faulty opinion

boiling point: The temperature at which a substance in liquid form boils and turns to vapor

capillary: A very tiny blood vessel that can be either an artery or a vein

cause and effect: A text structure in which the cause of an event directly precedes the outcome of the event, or its effect

cell: The basic biological unit of all living things

cellular respiration: The process of cells burning oxygen to obtain energy and giving off carbon dioxide as a waste product

cell theory: A fundamental theory of biology whose three hypotheses are (1) that all living things on Earth are composed of cells; (2) that a cell is the basic unit of life; and (3) that all cells come from preexisting cells.

central nervous system: The part of the nervous system that includes the brain and spinal cord

ceruminous glands: Glands found in the ear canals that secrete a waxy substance to protect the ear canal and lubricate the eardrum

chemical change: A change in the composition of atoms or molecules as a result of a chemical reaction; for example, when H_2O is broken into H_2 and O_2, the composition of atoms has changed

chromosomes: Structures in the cell nucleus that are made up of DNA and contain the genetic code for an organism; humans have 23 pairs of chromosomes

circuit: An electrical system in which current flows in a circular path

circulatory system: The body system that includes the heart and blood vessels

claim-evidence: Text structure in which a claim is stated and evidence is presented to support the claim

clause: A group of words that include a noun and a verb

colon: The punctuation mark (:) that typically introduces a list

comma: The punctuation mark (,) that signals a pause in the text

comma splice: A construction that combines two sentences into a single sentence separated by a comma; comma splices are not found in well-written text

command: A sentence that gives an order or makes a request

compare and contrast: A text structure in which an item is introduced in one section and then compared with another item in the following section

compound: A pure substance such as methane (CH_4) or water (H_2O), that is made up of two or more elements

concentration: The amount of solute that is dissolved in a solution; a solution with a high concentration has a large amount of solute dissolved

conclusion: A judgment or decision that a reader reaches from reading a text

constant: In algebra, a number that is not linked to a variable

context: The text that surrounds a particular item or passage and gives it background meaning

context clues: Hints about the meaning of a text that are derived from assessing its surrounding words, or context

control: A variable kept constant during an experiment

coordinating conjunction: The words that include *and, so, but, for, or, nor,* and *yet;* they are used to connect two independent clauses

coronal plane: Anatomical plane that divides body into front and back portions

covalent bonds: Chemical bonds in which electrons are shared equally

dash: A long dash (—) sets off important information in a sentence or introduces surprise; a short dash (–) connects numbers such as in "the period 1965–1968"

decimal: A number expressed in place values based on powers of 10

declarative: A sentence that states a fact or makes a statement

dendrites: The parts of a neuron that receive input from other neurons

denominator: The bottom part of a fraction

denotative meaning: The dictionary meaning of a word

density: Measures the amount of mass a substance has per unit volume

dependent clause: A clause that cannot stand on its own; for example, the italicized words in the following sentence comprise a dependent clause: *When the rain stopped,* Jo went home.

dependent variable: What an experiment measures as an effect or outcome

dermis: Middle layer of the skin, consisting of dense connective tissue

diabetes: A disease in which the body does not secrete a sufficient amount of insulin into the bloodstream; thus, body cells become "starved" because they cannot take in glucose

diameter: The distance across a circle through its center

difference: The answer in subtraction; in 9 – 4 = 5, the 5 is the difference

diffusion: The process in which material flows from a more concentrated area (e.g., in a solution) to an area that is less concentrated

digestive system: The body system that breaks down food and delivers it to the bloodstream

displacement: A change of position, typically the result of movement

divisor: In division, the number that divides into a second number; for 24 ÷ 3, the number 3 is the divisor

DNA: The genetic molecule that makes up chromosomes in the cells and forms the genetic code; DNA transmits information for the proteins that help carry out all important life processes

dominant: In genetics, an allele with a trait that prevails when it is present and the other allele is recessive; for example, a *tall* allele is dominant over a *short* allele

double replacement: A chemical reaction in which two components switch places as in *AB + CD → AD + CB*

drawing a conclusion: Using evidence and reasoning in a text to make a deduction

electric current: The movement of electrons

electronegativity: The tendency of an atom to attract electrons

electrons: Negatively charged fundamental particles that exist outside of the nucleus of every atom

element: A substance, such as carbon, nickel, or chlorine, that is made of a single type of atom

embryo: A growing organism that is incomplete and unborn

endocrine: Pertaining to hormones that secrete internally into the blood

endothermic: A change in state of matter that requires heat

energy: The ability to do work

entertain: One of the four purposes for which an author writes a text, which include to explain, persuade, entertain, or express feelings

enzyme: A protein that facilitates a chemical reaction

epidermis: Outermost layer of the skin

estimate: In math, to find an approximate answer

exclamatory: A sentence that expresses excitement or surprise

excretory system: The body system that removes cellular waste that is expelled from the body after being processed in the kidneys

exothermic: A change in state of matter that gives off heat

experiment: A scientific procedure to test a hypothesis or answer a question

explain: One of the four purposes for which an author writes a text, which include to explain, persuade, entertain, or express feelings

expository: A sentence or passage that explains

express feelings: One of the four purposes for which an author writes a text, which include to explain, persuade, entertain, or express feelings

fact: A description that can be supported by logic and evidence

factor: A quantity that when multiplied by another quantity equals a third quantity; 3 and 5 are both factors of 15 because $3 \times 5 = 15$

fertilization: The process in human reproduction in which the sperm penetrates the egg, the sperm and ovum nuclei fuse, and a zygote is formed

first person: A sentence told from the "I" or "me" point of view

footnote: An explanatory note keyed to the text and found at the bottom of the page

fractions: Division expressed in rational form with a numerator over a denominator

freezing point: The temperature at which a substance in liquid form becomes solid

fungi: Plantlike organisms (e.g., mushrooms, mold) that get their food from decaying material or other living things

gas: The state of matter in which atoms or molecules move freely and fill up any space that they inhabit

gas exchange: The process by which oxygen is delivered to the body cells and carbon dioxide is removed as waste

GCF (greatest common factor): The factor of two numbers that is greatest in value; the GCF of 8 and 12 is 4 because 4 is the greatest number that divides equally into both 8 and 12

gene: A section of a chromosome; typically a gene code for a particular protein

genotype: The genetic makeup of an organism with regard to its alleles; an organism with dominant and recessive "T" and "S" genes might have genotype TtSs, or ttSs, among others

glomerulus: A functional unit of the kidney that controls excretion

heart cycle: The rhythmic contraction and relaxation of heart muscles

homeostasis: The tendency of an organism to find a safe, stable state for all body functions within its internal environment

hormones: Chemicals that are secreted by glands, distributed through the blood, and facilitate activity and change in other parts of the body

host: An organism—animal or plant— that provides biological refuge for another—frequently parasitic—organism

hypertonic: An area in which matter is concentrated and tends to diffuse to a less concentrated area

hyphen: The small, dash-like punctuation mark (-) used to join words that are used as modifiers, such as the mark that joins "dash-like" here

hypodermis: Innermost layer of the skin that connects to underlying muscle and bone

hypothesis: A proposed explanation for a scientific phenomenon that can be tested in an experiment

hypotonic: An area in which a substance is less concentrated; a substance tends to diffuse into a hypotonic area from an area of higher concentration

idiom: A colloquial metaphor, such as "raining cats and dogs"

immune system: A network of cells, tissues, and organs that work in concert to protect the body from attack by tiny organisms that cause infections

improper fraction: A fraction in which the numerator is greater than the denominator

independent clause: A clause that can stand on its own as a complete sentence; in the following sentence, both clauses are independent: Ralph was hungry, so he bought a sandwich.

independent variable: What an experiment measures as a cause

inequality: A mathematical statement that two expressions are unequal

infectious diseases: Illnesses caused by microbes, or germs (e.g., bacteria, viruses, and fungi) that enter the body and multiply

inference: An educated guess that a reader makes about a text based on evidence within the text, logic, and personal experience

ingredients label: A label on a food product that reveals the food's nutritional composition

insulin: A hormone secreted by the pancreas that makes it possible for blood glucose to enter body cells

integers: Whole numbers that are both positive and negative and include zero

integumentary system: Organ system that consists of skin, hair, nails, glands, and nerves

interrogative: A sentence that asks a question

inverse operations: Mathematical operations that undo each other, such as addition and subtraction

ionic bond: A chemical bond between ions such as Na^+ and Cl^- in which the negative ion completely "captures" the electron from the positive ion

ionization energy: The energy required to remove an atom's outermost electron

ions: Atoms that take on extra electrons or give up an electron; ions typically exist in solution such as NaCl breaking up into Na^+ and Cl^- ions in water

isotopes: Atom species that contain a particular number of neutrons and therefore have particular atomic mass; isotopes of carbon include C^{14} and C^{12}

killer T cells: Cells in the immune system that kill off foreign cells in the body that are identified by helper cells

kingdom: One of the six divisions of biological organisms that include bacteria, archaeobacteria, plants, animals, fungi, and protists

large intestine: The lower portion of the body's digestive system that concentrates waste and delivers it so it can be expelled from the body

LCD (lowest common denominator): The lowest value that each individual denominator can divide into evenly; for example, 24 is the LCD for 5/12 and 3/8 because 24 is the lowest number that can be used as a denominator for both fractions: $5/12 = 10/24$; $3/8 = 9/24$

LCM (least common multiple): The lowest value that each of two or more values can divide into evenly; for example, 24 is the LCM for 12 and 8 because 24 is the lowest number that is a multiple of 12 and 8

like terms: Algebraic terms that have the same variable to the same power and can be combined using addition or subtraction

liquid: The state of matter in which particles are attracted but still can move somewhat freely

litmus paper: Paper used to determine the pH (acidity) of a chemical; blue litmus paper turns red in an acid and red litmus paper turns blue in a base

lungs: Organs in the human body used for breathing, taking in oxygen and expelling carbon dioxide

magnitude: The relative size of a substance or object that helps determine the appropriate measuring unit

main idea: The primary point in a text; the reason that a text is written

mean: The average of all the values in a data set

measures of central tendency: Statistical tools (mean, median, mode) that describe the trend of data

median: The middle point in a dataset, such that half of the data points are smaller and half of the data points are larger. The median doesn't have to be a member of the data set

meiosis: A type of cell division in which gametes (egg and sperm cells) are formed that have only a single set ($1n$) of chromosomes rather than the normal double ($2n$) set of chromosomes that all other body cells have

melting point: The temperature at which a substance in solid form becomes liquid

Mendel, Gregor: Considered the "father of modern genetics," a 19th-century scientist who was the first to propose a way in which traits are passed from one generation to the next, sometimes skipping generations

mental math: Calculation process that is carried out mentally without paper, pencil, or a mechanical or electronic calculating device

mitosis: Process in which cells divide to grow

mixture: A blend of particles

mode: The most common value in a data set; a data set can have more than one mode

molarity: The number of moles of a chemical per liter of solution; a solution of $2M$ contains 2 moles of the chemical for every liter of solution

mole: 6.02×10^{23} particles of a substance; for example, a mole of carbon has 6.02×10^{23} atoms and a mass of exactly 12 grams; a mole of oxygen has 6.02×10^{23} molecules and a mass of exactly 32 grams

molecule: The smallest particle of a substance that consists of atoms that are bonded to one another; for example, water consists of molecules of H_2O; nitrogen consists of molecules of N_2

musculoskeletal system: Body system that includes the muscles and bones and makes movement possible

mutation: A mistake in the copying of DNA that usually results in faulty proteins that are lethal but can sometimes result in beneficial adaptations

narrative: A text that has a story form

negative number: Any number that is less than zero

nephrons: Units of the excretory system within the kidney

neurons: Nerve cells

neurotransmitters: Chemicals released in a synapse that transmits an electrical nerve signal from one neuron to the next neuron

neutrons: Particles in the nucleus of an atom that have a mass of 1 amu but no charge

noun: A word that names a person, place, thing, or idea

nucleus: (1) Center part of an atom that contains protons and neutrons; (2) In a cell, the part of the cell that contains chromosomes and DNA

number line: Continuous line that includes all numbers, mainly used as an aid in inequalities, addition, and subtraction

numerator: Top part of a fraction

operation: Addition, subtraction, multiplication, or division

opinion: A statement that reflects a person's personal judgment, which may or may not be supported by evidence or facts

order of operations: Order in algebra in which operations are carried out, namely, parentheses, exponents, multiplication and division, addition and subtraction (abbreviated PEMDAS)

organ: Highly specialized body part such as the heart, brain, or liver that performs a specific function or group of functions

organelles: Discrete structures in cells such as mitochondria, the nucleus, Golgi bodies, and chloroplasts

organic: Chemical that contains carbon

ovaries: Female organs that produce eggs

parallel: Two lines that never meet

participle: A form of a verb that indicates an action or past action (called a past participle) and can also be used as an adjective; for example, the word *broiled* in "I ate broiled fish" is a participle used as an adjective, and the word *eaten* in "I have eaten" is a past participle

passive voice: A sentence or text in which the initiator of the action is not clearly identified; for example, *Mistakes were made*

pathogen: A microorganism (e.g., bacterium, virus) with the potential to cause disease or illness in its host

percentage: A special ratio that compares a quantity to 100

period: Punctuation mark (.) that ends a declarative sentence

periodic table: In chemistry, the table that organizes all 118 known elements into groups with similar properties

peristalsis: Muscular process by which food in the digestive system is moved through the system

personal pronoun: Pronoun that stands for a person, such as *I, you,* or *she*

persuasive: The type of writing that attempts to convince the reader to take a position or do something

pH: Log scale that measures the acidity of a substance; whereas low pH indicates high acidity, high pH indicates low acidity (highly basic)

phenotype: The body form of an organism as opposed to its genotype; when T is dominant for "tall," an individual with "tall" phenotype may have genotype TT or Tt

phrase: A group of words that does not include both a subject or predicate

physical changes: Changes that do not involve a change in chemical composition; ice melting is a physical change because H_2O does not change chemical composition during melting

place value: Value of a place in the number system; the 4 in the number 846 shows 4 in the *tens* column

possessive pronoun: Pronoun that shows possession such as *hers, yours,* or *mine*

predicate: The "verb" part of a sentence that expresses action or being

prediction: A guess made by the reader about future events or actions

prefix: A word part added to the beginning of a root or word to change its meaning

preposition: A word before a noun to show the relationship of the noun to another word or phrase in the sentence; examples include *for, in, at, from*

present participle: The verb form used with helping verbs (for example, *are* or *am*) that show ongoing action as *eating, bringing,* or *hearing*

primary source: A source created at the time period being studied, such as a letter, diary or original photograph

problem-solution: Text structure in which problems are posed and are followed by solutions

product: The answer in multiplication; in $4 \times 9 = 36$, the 36 is the product

pronoun: A word such as *he, she, it,* or *me* that takes the place of a noun

proper noun: A noun that names a person, place, or thing that is always capitalized, such as *Arizona* and *Donald Draper*

proportion: Special algebraic equation in which two ratios are set equal to one another

protein: Body chemicals that perform an enormous number of disparate functions, some of which are structural; many proteins function as enzymes that facilitate otherwise "impossible" chemical reactions that allow life processes such as metabolism to be carried out

protons: Positive particles in the nucleus of an atom that have atomic mass of 1 amu

protozoa: One-celled organisms that carry out complex metabolic activities; protozoa can be found nearly everywhere on Earth, and several protozoan parasites can cause serious diseases of the respiratory tract and the central nervous system

quotation marks: Punctuation (") that identifies the exact words of a speaker

quotient: The answer in division; in $40 \div 5 = 8$, the 8 is the quotient

radius: The distance from the center of a circle to any point on the circle

ratio: Relationship between two numbers that can be expressed in several ways; for example, as a fraction $\frac{4}{5}$, or as 4 to 5, 4:5

recessive: In genetics, a trait that is expressed only when *both* alleles are identical and recessive; for example, if *T* is dominant for tall and *t* is recessive for short, a *Tt* individual is tall, and only a *tt* individual is short

reciprocal: The result of a fraction in which the numerator and denominator of the original fraction switch places

red bone marrow: Consists of blood stem cells and blood cells in various stages of development

reliability: The probability that a scientific procedure or experiment or other procedure is repeatable

respiration: The process by which oxygen is used to break down food (e.g., sugar) and produce energy in the form of adenosine triphosphate (ATP) molecules

RNA: In cells, nucleic acids that carry out protein synthesis, expressing the code inscribed in DNA

rounding: In math, approximating a number to a certain place value; for example, 48 rounded to the nearest ten is 50

run-on: A construction that contains two independent clauses that should be broken up into two separate sentences

sagittal plane: Anatomical plane that divides body into left and right portions

sebaceous glands: Glands that produce sebum, an oily secretion that lubricates the skin and makes it more elastic

secondary source: A source that analyzes an event after it has happened—sometimes long afterward

second person: A sentence presented in terms of *you*

semicolon: A punctuation mark (;) that is used to separate independent clauses that are not connected by a conjunction or to separate items in a list

sentence: A group of words that includes a subject and predicate and expresses a complete thought

sentence fragment: A sentence-like construction that is incomplete in some way and therefore does not qualify as a sentence; typically, it is missing a subject or a predicate

sequence: A text structure that can take the form of a list, numbered steps, a bulleted list, or a series in outline form

series: A group of items that are connected in some consecutive way

sidebar: A sentence or short paragraph located at the side of the main text or in a box

sign: The designation of a number as positive (+) or negative (−)

simple sentence: A sentence that contains only a subject and a verb and has no clauses or phrases

simplest terms: A fraction with both numerator and denominator having their smallest possible values, but retaining the original fraction's value

single replacement: A chemical reaction in which one component switches for another as in AB + C → AC + B

slang: Informal language that is nonstandard and usually not appropriate in formal writing

slope: The ratio of rise to run in a graph calculated by the ratio of Δy to Δx; a graph with a high positive slope appears to rise sharply from left to right

small intestine: Part of the body's digestive system in which food is broken down into its smallest form and absorbed into the bloodstream

solid: State of matter in which particles are "frozen" into place and cannot move freely past one another

solubility: How readily a substance dissolves

solute: The substance that dissolves in a solution; in salt water, salt is the solute

solution: (1) A homogeneous mixture in which solute particles such as salt completely disappear within the solvent (e.g., water); (2) the answer to a math problem

solvent: The medium in a solution; in salt water, water is the solvent

standard anatomical position: The reference point for viewing the body to allow for consistent medical descriptions. For humans, standard anatomical position means standing up straight with the body at rest

stereotype: An oversimplified and often incorrect view of a group or a member of a group; for example, "hardworking" is a common stereotype for Asians

subject: The item that a phrase or a sentence is about

sudoriferous glands: Sweat glands that secrete water and sodium chloride and serve to cool the body's temperature

suffix: A word part added to the end of a root or word to change its meaning

sum: The answer in math when quantities are added; in 2 + 3 = 5, the 5 is the sum

summarizing: A brief, condensed accounting of a longer text

supporting detail: A fact or item within a text that supports a main idea

synonym: A word that has the same meaning or nearly the same meaning as another word

synthesis: Process in which two (or more) items are combined to form a single item

testosterone: Male sex hormone

text structure: Text that has a particular format such as sequence, problem–solution, or cause and effect

theme: A text's highest and most general subject; the message the author wants to get across

third person: Text written from the "he," "she," and "they" points of view

tissues: Cells that are joined together for a single function, such as muscle tissue

topic: The subject of a text

topic sentence: Sentence that typically contains the main idea of a paragraph

transverse plane: Anatomical plane that divides body into top and bottom portions

triple point: The temperature and pressure at which all three states of matter can exist at once

unlike terms: Algebraic terms that cannot be combined using addition or subtraction because they do not share the same variable to the same power

uterus: Part of the female reproductive system in which fertilized eggs implant and grow into embryos, eventually developing into fetuses

vaccine: A weakened form of an antigen that is deliberately introduced into the body to activate the production of antibodies to prevent disease

valence electrons: The outermost electrons in an atom that are typically lost or gained when the atom forms an ion

validity: Ability of a scientific procedure or experiment to measure a specific quantity or quality

variable: In algebra, a letter quantity that can stand for any number or quantity

veins: Blood vessels that carry blood to the heart; typically, veins carry deoxygenated blood, but the pulmonary vein that goes from the lungs to the heart carries oxygenated blood

ventricles: The lower chambers of the heart

verb: An action word or a word of being; for example, *run, eat,* or *is*

virus: A nonliving infectious microbe that is a chain of nucleic acids (DNA or RNA); it lives in a host cell, replicating via cellular mechanisms

viscosity: Measures a substance's resistance to motion when subjected to an applied force

volts: A measurement of energy in a battery or electrical system; a system with greater voltage has greater electrical "pressure" for electrons to move and current to flow

volume: Measures the amount of space a substance occupies

zygote: A fertilized egg that has not yet begun to divide